Ro
is
Bo

Overcoming Common Problems Series

Selected titles

A full list of titles is available from Sheldon Press,
36 Causton Street, London SW1P 4ST and on our website at
www.sheldonpress.co.uk

Overcoming Common Problems Series

Overcoming Common Problems Series

Overcoming Common Problems

The Irritable Bowel Diet Book

Second edition

ROSEMARY NICOL

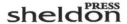

First published in Great Britain in 1990

Sheldon Press
36 Causton Street
London SW1P 4ST
www.sheldonpress.co.uk

Reprinted eleven times
Second edition published 2013

The author and publisher have made every effort to ensure that the external website and email addresses included in this book are correct and up to date at the time of going to press. The author and publisher are not responsible for the content, quality or continuing accessibility of the sites.

British Library Cataloguing-in-Publication Data
A catalogue record for this book is available from the British Library

ISBN 978-1-84709-302-8
eBook ISBN 978-1-84709-303-5

Typeset by Caroline Waldron, Wirral, Cheshire
First printed in Great Britain by Ashford Colour Press
Subsequently digitally printed in Great Britain

Produced on paper from sustainable forests

Contents

Acknowledgements

The publisher would like to acknowledge the help given by the following people for the new edition of this book:

Dr Jenny Lee, Senior Dietitian, and other members of the Gastroenterology Department at Addenbrooke's Hospital, Cambridge University Hospitals NHS Foundation Trust.

Glutafin for recipes from their web page <www.glutafin.co.uk> as follows: white bread (page 57), warm Italian flatbread (page 57), brown bread (page 57), fibre oven-baked loaf (page 58).

I would like to acknowledge the help given to me by the following people:

Mr Andrew Gough, Consultant Surgeon, Weston General Hospital, Weston-super-Mare; Dr Ken Heaton, Reader in Medicine, University of Bristol Department of Medicine; Professor John Hunter, Consultant Physician, and Mrs Elizabeth Workman, Research Dietitian, Gastroenterology Research Department, Addenbrooke's Hospital, Cambridge; Tesco Supermarket, Weston-super-Mare.

From *The Gluten-free and Wheat-free Bumper Bake Book*, by Rita Greer (1982): shortcrust pastry (page 59), crispbreads (page 59), banana bread (page 60), basic plain cake and flavourings (page 63), basic fruit cake (page 63), rich chocolate cake (page 64), plain biscuits and flavourings (page 64), ginger nuts (page 65). From *Healthier Special Diets* by Rita Greer (1987), chapatis (page 61), tortillas (page 62), tacos (page 62), fruit cookies (page 65), pancake batter (page 53).

I thank the following publishers for permission to reprint recipes from their books as follows: Macdonald for date and walnut loaf (page 60), simple banana loaf (page 61) and homemade baking powder (page 62) from *The Food Intolerance Diet Book*, by Elizabeth Workman, Dr Virginia Alun Jones and Dr John Hunter (1986); and Century Arrow for buckwheat loaf (page 60) and pancakes (page 53) from *Wheat and Gluten-free Cookery*, by Judy Ridgway (1986).

Note to the reader

This is not a medical book and is not intended to replace advice from your doctor. Consult your pharmacist or doctor if you believe you have any of the symptoms described, and if you think you might need medical help.

1

What is irritable bowel syndrome?

Take your mind back to the last time you went out to a social function. Imagine yourself, plate and glass in hand, passing gracefully among interesting people, enjoying witty, intelligent conversation. What did you talk about? The weather? The political situation? Your job? Your holidays? Your bowels?

> 'Good evening, I've been so looking forward to meeting you. Do tell me all about your latest bowel movements. More salad?'
>
> 'Just a small helping, please. Well, I've been particularly constipated this week. Can I pass you the potatoes?'
>
> 'Thank you, I'd love some. Now my problem is diarrhoea. You wouldn't believe how many times I had to go yesterday – ten and that's the truth.'
>
> 'Well I never! Isn't that quiche just too delicious?'
>
> 'Absolute perfection. Yes, my stools have been most interesting lately. On Monday . . .'

At this stage you move quickly out of earshot, having suddenly lost your appetite.

In reality, of course, it wouldn't be like that at all. As a race we have been brought up not to discuss, or even think about, anything to do with bowels or bowel movements. This is a pity, because we all have bowel movements and what could be more normal or healthy than passing out of the body the waste products of the food we eat?

Unfortunately if you have irritable bowel syndrome (IBS) there are times when you may not feel either normal or healthy. In fact, IBS might so upset your life that you would avoid going to the sort of social function where you would need to pass among gracious people making witty conversation as you eat food cooked to perfection. Diarrhoea and the need to remain near a toilet may play havoc with your social life and your self-confidence. Or you may be so constipated you feel constantly bloated, uncomfortable and full of wind.

If you have irritable bowel syndrome, take comfort. You are not alone. The chances are that about one in five of the people you know get it, though they may not talk about it. At one extreme are healthy robust individuals who don't go to the doctor about it and don't feel it upsets their lives in any way; they get it from time to time, but it hardly bothers them. At the other extreme are those for whom IBS is devastating. They daren't move far from a toilet; they feel isolated, panicky, totally lacking in self-confidence. Their social life is ruined, their diet is badly restricted, and they worry that their ill-health may cause them to lose their job. Their tummy becomes the centre of the universe, and they live in fear of the tricks their body may have in store for them. In between are the great majority, who manage quite well most of the time, but still have to watch what they eat, and find their gut plays them up if they get tense or agitated.

If you have read my book *Coping Successfully with Your Irritable Bowel*, I hope you will have overcome any natural embarrassment concerning bodily functions, their names and their descriptions. For those of you who have not read it, it deals with all aspects of irritable bowel syndrome – its causes, its many and varied symptoms, the problems of diagnosis, the range of medical investigations and treatments, abdominal pain, constipation, diarrhoea, stress, the relationship between IBS and your personality and upbringing, the role of alternative medicine – and much more. There is also a chapter especially for women.

IBS is not a disease – it is a disorder of the way part of the digestive system works and of how it reacts to certain things like food and stress. It is a condition which comes and goes, it is tiresome and extremely common, but it is not life-threatening, it is not cancer or related in any way to cancer, nor it is any form of serious bowel disease.

The main symptoms of IBS are:

- abdominal pain (that is, pain in the tummy), usually low down on the left, or possibly centre or right;
- diarrhoea, with or without stomach pain;
- constipation, usually with stomach pain, and small lumpy stools like 'rabbit droppings';
- alternating diarrhoea and constipation, often in an unpredictable and erratic fashion;
- an abdomen that looks or feels bloated and distended;
- feeling 'full of wind';
- passing mucus with the stools, or by itself;

- in addition it generally becomes worse during periods of stress, and may disappear completely at other times.

There are also a whole number of other bowel, bladder, digestive, emotional and physical symptoms – all of which are quite common in IBS. Bear in mind that IBS affects the whole length of the gut (it used to be thought it only affected the colon), thus increasing the possibility of a whole range of symptoms. For example, some people feel tired all the time. IBS can also cause back pain and gynaecological symptoms such as pain during or after intercourse. One study found 50 per cent of women seeking help for pain during intercourse had the syndrome. Some women notice that their IBS becomes worse during their period, it is thought because of prostaglandins secreted from the uterus.

Red-flag symptoms

Although IBS can be uncomfortable, there are certain warning or 'red-flag' symptoms that you should not accept as being just part of the condition. The symptoms below are usually associated with organic diseases such as Crohn's disease and ulcerative colitis, or possibly a more serious illness such as bowel cancer, so always see your GP if you experience:

- passing blood with your stools, or rectal bleeding – 25 per cent of people with IBS experience this because of straining, but it should always be checked out;
- unexplained weight loss;
- being awakened by IBS-like symptoms;
- fever;
- start of IBS symptoms or any rapid and persistent unexplained change in bowel habits if you are over 40.

Many people with IBS say that it becomes worse during periods of stress. Others connect it solely with what they eat. Some can find nothing at all that triggers it. Even doctors are not in complete agreement, some believing it is 'all in the mind', others that it is usually caused by an intolerance to one or more foods, others that it results from stress, or a combination of all these.

Most people can trace their IBS back to a period of stress (which can affect the way food is propelled through the digestive system), or to

Ovarian cancer symptoms and IBS symptoms

Department of Health guidelines now stress that GPs should look for early signs of ovarian cancer, which are often confused with those of IBS. Unlike IBS symptoms, though, which may come and go, ovarian cancer symptoms tend to be more persistent and to have no obvious trigger such as food. The cancer charity Target Ovarian Cancer highlights three key factors in symptoms – they are:

- frequent (more than 12 times a month);
- persistent (they don't go away);
- new – they are not normal for you and may have started in the last year.

Key symptoms to be aware of are:

- Persistent pelvic or abdominal pain
- Increased abdominal size/persistent bloating – not bloating that comes and goes
- Difficulty eating or feeling full quickly
- Urinary symptoms (needing to pass water more urgently or more often than usual).

Changes in bowel habit, extreme fatigue, unexplained weight loss and loss of appetite should also be taken seriously.

Ovarian cancer affects mainly post-menopausal women, and is rare in women under 40. It is the fifth most common cancer in the UK – 7,000 women a year are diagnosed with ovarian cancer (as opposed to around 50,000 women with breast cancer, say). So, while comparatively uncommon, it is still worth keeping an eye out for. Do discuss any worrying symptoms with your doctor.

a bout of gastroenteritis – 'holiday tummy' – (which may make the intestines over-reactive and sensitive), or to a long course of antibiotics (which may affect the delicate balance of beneficial bacteria in the gut), or to an abdominal or pelvic operation (especially if you had a course of antibiotics beforehand). Whatever triggered it for you, the chances are that stress and some foods make it worse.

If food is your problem, I hope that by the end of this book you will have a better understanding of why your gut reacts to some foods the way it does, and will feel able to eat a balanced interesting diet without upsetting your insides.

2

One man's wheat . . .
a look at problem foods

There is now evidence to suggest that intolerance to specific foods – as distinct from allergy – is common, and may be an important factor in the aetiology [cause] of the irritable bowel syndrome.

(Lessof 1983)

Approximately 50 per cent of the patients attending a gastroenterology clinic have IBS, and 50 per cent of those patients can be managed by elimination diets. That must reflect a huge potential saving of long-term cost by the patient and of course long-term saving by the NHS exchequer. The patient can then take charge of their own disease.

(Professor Jonathan Brostoff, *Foods Matter*, no date)

Two hundred patients (156 women) with irritable bowel syndrome were treated with dietary exclusion for three weeks. Nearly half (48.2 per cent) showed symptomatic improvement. Subsequent challenge with individual foods showed that around three-quarters of these responders were able to identify one or more food intolerances. The majority identified two to five foods which upset them. The foods most commonly incriminated were dairy products (40.7 per cent) and grains (39.4 per cent).

(R. Nanda et al. 1989)

Evidence for a physical cause for IBS should come as a relief for those of you who've been castigating yourselves as hypochondriacs – or been at the receiving end of others' castigation. While a certain amount of somatisation (psychological distress expressed as physical symptoms) is thought to play a part in some cases of IBS, many experts agree that we must first look for hidden physical causes of IBS before treating psychological factors associated with the condition. Among these, research suggests that food sensitivities are often a clear and well-defined common cause.

Not all in the head

There's still a myth that IBS is a psychological condition. But, while stress can undoubtedly make symptoms worse, there is growing evidence that more than half of those with IBS have a food intolerance that often develops after a bout of food poisoning or gastroenteritis that leaves the gut hypersensitive. As a result, the gut reacts slightly differently, with changes in gut bacteria that make them respond to low-grade inflammation with abnormal fermentation.

Clinical studies from the departments of gastroenterology at the John Radcliffe Hospital in Oxford and Addenbrooke's Hospital in Cambridge have shown that food is implicated in 50 per cent of patients with IBS (and also Crohn's) and that the reactions are specific and confirmed by double-blind food challenges. Elimination of the culprit food can clear up not only symptoms in the gut but more general symptoms as well. In one study, researchers at Cambridge University found that IBS patients eating a normal diet produced large amounts of hydrogen, but that an exclusion diet relieved excess gas and other IBS symptoms.

In particular, *the gut lining* has been pinpointed as the arbiter of reactions to foods – like a delicate sensor that reacts to culprit foods. In 2010, a research team of biologists led by Professor Michael Schemann at the Technische Universitaet Muenchen (TUM) found that mini-inflammations of the gut lining upset the sensitive balance of the bowel and cause sensitisation of the digestive nervous system, so leading to IBS (Science News 2010). In other words, IBS can be the result of low-level inflammation of the gut wall. 'The irritated gut mucosa produces increased amounts of neuroactive substances such as serotonin, histamine and protease. This cocktail produced by the body could be the real cause of the unpleasant IBS complaints,' says Professor Schemann.

Debate still continues as to whether the causes of IBS are primarily physical or mental but it is increasingly being recognised that they may be a complex interweaving of both. There is a great deal of continuing research into the gut as a second brain, and how they interact – or neurogastroenterology. Incidentally, this throws light on why people with IBS are often prescribed antidepressants – it's thought that antidepressants work on the many nerves in the gut, with low-dose tricyclic antidepressants among the most effective treatments. Some doctors do view IBS as among the symptoms of clinical depression – but those with IBS are often unhappy because of their debilitating symptoms. Professor Jonathan Brostoff is a well-known advocate of IBS being caused by diet, not the mind, in many IBS patients, with allergy and infection as associated causes. 'Of course we need to treat the whole patient and as the brain (in the skull) is hard wired to the "brain" of the gut, it would hardly be surprising if the one did not affect the other,' says Professor Brostoff.

The commonest foods to cause IBS are wheat and milk, although usually people find problems with one or the other, not both. Of those whose IBS is caused by food intolerance, nearly half can trace it to wheat or milk.

Coffee, corn and onion come next, affecting 20–25 per cent, with chocolate, citrus fruits (oranges, lemons, limes, grapefruit), eggs, potatoes, oats, tea, yeast, barley and rye causing problems to 10–18 per cent. A number of other foods affect fewer than 10 per cent.

Wheat and milk are the most common foods eaten in Western countries; most of us eat them every day and usually in every meal and snack in some form or other. It could just be the fact that they are consumed so often that causes such widespread intolerance; it is probably true that very few people have problems with, say, cloves, salsify or pinto beans!

Intolerance to wheat

Intolerance to wheat is not the same thing as coeliac disease, which is caused by the inability of the intestine to absorb the gluten in wheat, rye, barley and oats. Coeliac disease can be identified by recognised medical tests, which IBS cannot.

However, because the two conditions are often confused, and because there is a certain degree of overlap between them, misdiagnosis can be a factor in both IBS and coeliac disease. It is also possible for both conditions to co-exist in the same person – research suggests that coeliac disease is four times as common in people with IBS as in the rest of the population. So, ideally, the possibility of coeliac disease needs to be ruled out before you go ahead with your new diet plans. Indeed, updated guidelines from the National Institute for Health and Care Excellence (NICE) with regard to IBS diagnosis state that coeliac disease must be ruled out by appropriate tests before a diagnosis of IBS can be made with confidence. So, if it is some time since your diagnosis of IBS was made, it is well worth revisiting this with your doctor.

Untreated coeliac disease may contribute to the development of a range of health problems including osteoporosis, osteopenia and certain kinds of cancer. It has also been linked with other disorders such as diabetes and thyroid disease. You should also ensure that any children with suspected IBS do not in fact have coeliac disease, as undiagnosed coeliac disease can cause growth or developmental problems. Again, consult your doctor if you suspect a child has coeliac disease.

For many with IBS, though, problems are caused by an intolerance to wheat, not an allergy to it, so there are no cut-and-dried medical tests (Chapter 3 has more about this). Why people may have wheat intolerance is not fully understood. Unlike coeliac disease, which is the inability to process gliadin, the protein found in gluten, intolerance may not involve gluten – although as the amount of wheat we consume rises, increasing numbers of people are reporting problems digesting wheat-based products.

Symptoms of wheat intolerance include bloating, headaches and joint pains. Some experts believe it occurs when some people are short of the enzymes necessary for the proper digestion of wheat. In any case, large portions of pasta and bread can also be hard to digest as they absorb water, swelling in the body and so causing discomfort. It may also be that wheat is wrongly blamed for intolerance, whereas the culprit is actually a dairy product such as the cheese sprinkled on pasta or used in a sandwich (don't forget that lactose intolerance is often confused with IBS – see page 10 for more on lactose intolerance).

If wheat is only a minor problem to you, you may be all right if you take it just once every few days. But if it causes serious IBS symptoms you will have to avoid all wheat flour – white, brown, granary and wholewheat. Substitutes are rice flour, potato flour, soya flour, rye flour, maize flour, millet flour and ground rice; or you could use buckwheat (no relation to wheat despite its name), millet, oats or oatmeal (see Appendix 2 for a list of substitute foods). Your local health food shop will probably stock some of these. All the substitute flours cook differently from wheat flour, so experiment before you use them instead of ordinary flour in recipes. Books on gluten-free cooking are available from libraries, online booksellers, bookshops and health food shops, as are books written specially for people with coeliac disease, and they contain recipes for substitute flours. The internet is a wonderful source of recipes for any medical condition.

Because wheat crops up in a wide variety of foods, you will need to read food labels carefully. Any of the following means that the product could contain wheat:

- wholegrain
- cereal protein
- wheatmeal
- cornflour
- flour
- edible starch
- starch
- food starch
- modified starch
- vegetable protein
- rusk
- thickening
- wheat protein
- thickener.

Many of the recipes in this book contain gluten-free flour. Most super-markets have 'free-from' shelves with flours and a wide range of other products suitable for people with food sensitivity. There is also a wide range of speciality outlets, including online shopping (see 'Useful addresses'). Sales of 'free-from' foods are soaring – in 2011, £230 million was spent on products like gluten-free bread and lactose-free milk in the UK and the overall market is now valued at an estimated £300 million as more people self-diagnose food sensitivities using online tools. Mintel anticipate that sales will reach £519 million by 2016. Yet when I first wrote this book in 1990, you had to order wheat-free flour from a specialist outlet or your pharmacy – or if you were excep-tionally lucky, they might have it tucked away on a shelf somewhere. Readers were unlikely to find what they needed on the supermarket shelves, and I advised them to write to the head office of their local supermarket, to see if they could send a list of suitable alternatives to products containing wheat or dairy. How times have changed! Now you're likely to spend almost as much time scanning the supermarket shelves for the best 'free-from' product as you would ever have done hunting down sources of suitable foods in the old days.

However, the human gut remains the same, so if you think you do have an allergy or intolerance, follow the advice in this chapter, and ask your doctor for help if need be. There are many good books on IBS and diet (see 'References and further reading'). One of my inspirations was the pioneering *The Gluten-free and Wheat-free Bumper Bake Book* by Rita Greer, a collection of over 300 recipes for biscuits, breads, party foods, packed meal ideas and nutritional advice. (You may be able to get hold of a copy through Amazon, eBay or Abe Books, or see 'References and further reading' for more suggestions.) I am grateful to Rita Greer for her permission to use some of these recipes in this book.

If you take no wheat or gluten for long periods you may get a deficiency of B-group vitamins – thiamine, riboflavin, nicotinic acid, folic acid, pyridoxine and vitamin B_{12}. Ask your doctor about vitamin B supplements.

Possible substitutes for some common wheat-based foods are:

Breakfast cereals	Rice Krispies, puffed rice, porridge, some makes of muesli
Bread and biscuits	rice cakes, rice crackers, oat cakes, rye breads and crispbreads, bread and biscuits made with non-wheat flour
Wheat flour	other flours previously listed (which may cook differently from wheat flour); also arrowroot, tapioca, sago, millet, buckwheat; thicken sauces with tapioca flour, potato flour, ground rice
Pasta	non-wheat pasta, rice, potatoes
Baking powder	mix together 35 g bicarbonate of soda, 70 g cream of tartar and 70 g of arrowroot. Store in an airtight container and use 1½ teaspoons of this baking powder for 1 teaspoon of ordinary baking powder.

Intolerance to dairy products

Milk contains a naturally occurring sugar called lactose, which is broken down during digestion by an enzyme called lactase. Some people do not produce enough lactase, so they can't properly break down the lactose in milk products, and this can lead to pain and diarrhoea. It is possible that people with IBS are more likely than other people to have this inability to break down lactose during digestion.

In addition, lactose intolerance is often mistaken for IBS – like coeliac disease, it's another of the differential diagnoses doctors are on the look-out for when diagnosing IBS (or should be). As many as one in ten people in the UK – and more among those of African or Asian descent – has lactose intolerance. Cut down on dairy products and see if your symptoms improve. You can also try supplements of lactase – the enzyme that digests lactose.

Like wheat, dairy products (milk, butter, cheese, yogurt and cream) are in a great many of the foods we eat, so check food labels carefully.

If the label mentions:

- whey
- whey solids
- casein
- lactic acid
- E270 (lactic acid), E325 (sodium lactate), E327 (calcium lactate) or E472 (b) (lactic acid esters)
- any form of the word 'milk'

that product contains a milk-based substance.

However, it is still perfectly possible to have a nutritious and fulfilling diet. Goat's or ewe's milk products will probably be all right, unless you have a serious allergy to all dairy products. Yogurts and most cheeses have much less lactose than milk and most people can take them, especially in small quantities. Heating milk to boiling point can change some of the substances that trigger unpleasant symptoms, and evaporated milk is fine for many people as its heat treatment destroys some of the milk proteins that cause problems.

If you really can't take any naturally occurring dairy products, soya milk is now widely available, and you will probably get used to it very quickly. It can be used as a substitute for milk in drinks, in cooking and on cereal. Try to use soya milk that has been fortified with calcium. You can make your own soya milk: mix 165 g (6 oz) soya into a paste with a small quantity of water, add 1 litre (1¾ pints) of water, bring slowly to the boil, then simmer for 20 minutes, stirring all the time. Store it in the fridge.

Most everyday soft margarines (including at least one brand of own-label 'soya margarine') contain whey, a milk by-product. Look for dairy-free substitutes such as supermarket own-brand free-from margarines, or sunflower spreads such as Vitalite or supermarket own-brands.

Substitutes that contain no dairy products are Granose and Tomor kosher brands, and also tahini (ground sesame seeds). Some people find ghee – clarified butter – suits them; you can make it by melting some butter gently over a low heat, allowing it to cool slightly, then pouring it carefully into another container, taking care to leave at the bottom of the saucepan the 'scum'-like granules which are the proteins that may cause problems to people who can't take dairy products. Keep it in the fridge. Ghee is available in most Indian grocery stores.

If you take little or no dairy products, you will need to replace milk's many important ingredients, especially calcium and vitamin A. Calcium is not easily available in any other form except supplement tablets, and is essential for the growth of bones and teeth, and for important bodily processes such as blood clotting. It is especially important for girls and young women to take enough calcium to reduce the risk of osteoporosis in later years, yet these are the very years when they might cut down on dairy products if they perceive them as fattening. Soya milk contains no calcium (unless you buy a brand that is calcium-fortified) so if in doubt ask your doctor about calcium supplements. The UK recommended daily amount (RDA) of calcium is currently 700 mg a day, and the current thinking is that more is not better, but again, do check with your doctor if you think you have a special need for extra calcium.

Intolerance to other foods

Irritable bowel syndrome is not the end of civilised eating as we know it. No matter what upsets your gut, there are substitute foods that are perfectly acceptable, and that you will almost certainly quickly get used to (see also Appendix 2):

Chocolate	Carob, cocoa
Coffee or tea	Herb teas, fruit juices, Barleycup, Bovril, Caro, chicory drinks
Citrus fruits	Almost any other fruit
Potatoes	Rice, pasta, pulses
Corn oil or vegetable oil	Sunflower or safflower or soyabean oil
Corn	Wheat, rye, oats, barley

If yeast is a problem, avoid alcoholic drinks, yeast spreads such as Marmite, bread (except soda bread or any unleavened bread), yogurt, commercial fruit juices, B-group vitamins unless labelled 'yeast-free' and hydrolysed vegetable protein.

FODMAPs and IBS

FODMAPs are a type of carbohydrate common in foods that can be difficult to digest, especially for those with IBS, and removing them from the diet has been shown to improve symptoms in 76 per cent of those with IBS. Found in common foods such as fruits, dairy products, vegetables and grains, FODMAPS (that's fermentable oligosaccharides, disaccharides, monosaccharides and polyols to you and me) are poorly absorbed in the small intestine, meaning that they move on undigested to the large intestine and colon, where bacteria will cause excess gas, bloating and changes in fluid balance.

The low FODMAP diet was pioneered by Dr Sue Shepherd in Australia and was developed by a team at Monash University in Melbourne. It has been successfully adapted to the UK by researchers at King's College London and implemented at Guy's and St Thomas' NHS Trust in London. People on the diet go for eight weeks without consuming any FODMAP-rich foods. As well as giving up familiar IBS culprits such as cabbage and beans, they must also give up, for example:

- foods containing excess fructose such as honey, apples, pears and watermelon;
- foods containing fructans such as wheat and onions;
- foods containing polyols found in stone fruits such as plums and peaches and cherries as well as in polyol sweeteners such as sorbitol, often added to sugar-free varieties of mint, chocolate and chewing gum.

See Table 2.1 overleaf for more detail on FODMAPs in foods.

The diet needs careful administration to ensure that it is nutritionally adequate and effective, and it's not recommended that people with IBS self-administer. It works best under the supervision of a specialist, FODMAP-trained dietitian – this is important not just when giving foods up but when re-introducing them. Sometimes people feel so much better for giving up certain foods they are reluctant to experiment with a diet that seems to be working, but nutritionists stress that it's important not to give up foods unnecessarily, to avoid nutrient shortages. So, if you are interested in FODMAPs, you should consult your GP – or, if you wish to see a private dietitian trained in FODMAPs, you can search at <www.freelancedietitians.org>, run by the British Dietetic Association's Freelance Dietitian Group. Otherwise, it may be simpler to follow an exclusion diet to see if you can identify particular foods which disagree with you, so do see the information about exclusion diets on page 26.

Table 2.1 FODMAPs in foods

Excess fructose	Honey, apples, mango, pear, watermelon, high fructose corn syrup, corn syrup solids
Fructans	Artichokes (globe and Jerusalem), asparagus, beetroot, chicory, dandelion leaves, garlic (in large amounts), leek, onion, wheat (in large amounts), rye (in large amounts), inulin, fructo-oligosaccharides
Lactose	Milk, ice cream, custard, dairy desserts, condensed and evaporated milk, milk powder, yoghurt, margarine, soft unripened cheeses (e.g. ricotta, cottage, cream, mascarpone)
Galacto-oligosaccharides (GOS)	Legume beans (e.g. baked beans, kidney beans, borlotti beans), lentils, chickpeas
Polyols	Apples, apricots, avocados, cherries, lychees, nectarines, pears , plums, prunes, mushrooms, sorbitol (E420), mannitol (E421), xylitol (E967), maltitol (E965) and isomalt (E953)

Adapted from Shepherd Works – for updates visit <http://shepherdworks.com.au/disease-information/low-fodmap-diet>.

3

Food allergy or food intolerance?

Have you ever wondered whether your IBS is caused by your allergy to certain foods? After all, there is no doubt that some foods can make the condition worse for many people. Is this due to an allergy to those foods?

Perhaps when you have asked your doctor whether you might be allergic to the foods that are giving you problems, he or she has dismissed the idea and told you that your IBS is 'all in the mind', and if only you worried less about it your gut would return to normal.

It is certainly true that for most people their IBS becomes worse when they are under stress, and my book *Coping Successfully with Your Irritable Bowel* has lots of suggestions for coping with stress. Do also have a look at page 32 where I describe the latest findings on gut-targeted hypnotherapy, which has achieved good results in those with IBS. But there are also many whose symptoms are triggered less by their state of mind than by what they eat. Of course, sometimes the two are linked: researchers have found that if you eat something you think will disagree with you, your anxiety about that food causes changes to take place in your body that disrupt the digestive process and cause the unpleasant reactions; so your state of mind can be causing your upset gut.

Or perhaps the very thought of having to eat out gets you worried. It is surprising how many people get IBS symptoms *before* they eat out, perhaps before they even leave the house. The symptoms are obviously not being caused by the food but simply by the worry of eating out.

There are four basic reactions to food:

1 You like it, and can eat it with no problems.
2 Food aversion – you dislike or avoid a particular food for purely psychological reasons; for example, you don't like to eat fat, or meat, or spicy or 'foreign' foods.
3 Food allergy.
4 Food intolerance.

This chapter is concerned with the last two – food allergy and food intolerance.

Food allergy

An allergy is an adverse reaction involving the body's immune system, and the response to whatever is causing it is usually immediate and can be severe. The substance that causes the reaction is called the 'allergen'. Common allergens are:

- pollens and grasses
- the house dust mite and its droppings
- fur and feathers
- some foods and food additives
- some ingredients of clothing, creams and cosmetics
- certain drugs, such as penicillin
- insect bites and stings.

Typical conditions caused by allergy are asthma, some forms of eczema, hay fever, rhinitis (a constant congested or runny nose) and urticaria (nettle rash). It is interesting that many people with the diarrhoeal form of irritable bowel syndrome also have one or more of these typical allergies. If you already have one of these conditions it is more likely that sensitivity to food is causing your abdominal symptoms, and a diet that improves your IBS may well improve your allergy condition too.

With an allergy you develop abnormal antibodies to the allergens, and the antibodies react against the allergen by producing chemicals such as histamines, which cause typical allergic symptoms like wheezing, a runny nose or a rash. Doctors often prescribe antihistamines to overcome these unpleasant symptoms.

There are well-recognized and reliable tests to identify individual allergens, the two most common being the skinprick test and the RAST test.

The skinprick test (SPT)

This is the standard test for allergy. A small extract of the suspected allergen is placed on the arm, and a prick or scratch is made in the skin below the drop so that a small amount of the allergen enters the skin. If the patient is sensitive to that allergen a noticeable reaction will appear on the skin. This test is not always conclusive one way or the other.

The RAST test (radioallergosorbent test)

This will usually follow a skinprick test. It measures the level of immunoglobulin E (IgE) antibodies that the patient has to a specific substance, and thereby the extent to which he or she is allergic to that substance.

An individual's response to an allergen usually lasts for many years, perhaps even a lifetime, and can be caused by tiny amounts of that allergen – in extreme cases, for example by being in the same house as a cat, or spreading bread with a knife on which is just a trace of butter. Food allergy has the same reactions as any other sort of allergy; when you develop antibodies against a particular food, the food becomes the allergen, and the antibodies combine with that food to cause the unpleasant symptoms.

Food intolerance

Food intolerance is rather different. It is an adverse reaction to food in which the involvement of the immune system is unproven because skinprick and other tests for allergy are negative. This doesn't mean that immune reactions aren't involved, but it is unlikely that they are the main cause of the symptoms. So far there is no single reliable test of food intolerance (but see Chapter 4 on the exclusion diet, page 26).

Some foods contain chemicals that upset some people, possibly by upsetting the balance of bacteria in the gut and producing chemicals that cause the symptoms to develop. Conditions thought to be caused, or made worse, by food intolerance are:

- constipation
- Crohn's disease
- diarrhoea
- fatigue
- hyperactivity in children
- irritable bowel syndrome
- joint pain
- migraine
- nausea
- stomach and duodenal ulcers
- vomiting.

Culprit foods tend to be those that are taken regularly (milk, wheat, coffee, onions, for example), which is one reason why it can be difficult to identify the cause, and also why many people cannot trace the start of the symptoms to a particular time; they usually just notice mild symptoms such as a headache, indigestion or an upset stomach that gradually gets worse over a period of time. To make diagnosis even harder, symptoms may come and go, get better for a while, then worse. Unlike food allergy, food intolerance may disappear if the offending food is avoided for several months and then taken only in small quantities, although it may recur if the food is eaten frequently.

While it is true that intolerances can come and go, it is also true that avoiding one staple food may increase the use of another, and this over-use can create a new sensitivity. The new food may not have bothered you when you took it only occasionally, but by taking it in large quantities you may develop an intolerance to it. Be cautious, therefore, about taking new foods too frequently. You may also develop new intolerances that are triggered by antibiotics, virus infections or gastroenteritis.

If you think your IBS is caused by allergy to any staple food like wheat or dairy products, ask your doctor to arrange an allergy test for you. If the test turns out to be negative, accept that you are not allergic to the food but that you may well have an intolerance to it, so eat less of it, worry less about eating it, perhaps even avoid having it for several months and then introduce it in small quantities.

Not being able to eat what you like can be inconvenient, and having to avoid basic foods can lead to a disrupted lifestyle, a diminished social life and even under-nutrition. So don't jump to instant conclusions about what does or doesn't agree with you. Although a few people find that many foods trigger their IBS symptoms, most find they can manage quite well by avoiding just two or three. If you have any doubt about your diet talk to your general practitioner or a dietitian.

An audit of 1,000 patients at Addenbrooke's Hospital in Cambridge, led by senior consultant gastroenterologist Dr Stephen Middleton, found that dietary treatment was successful in over 70 per cent of patients. This suggests that almost three-quarters of those with IBS can prevent, or at least greatly reduce, the number and severity of attacks through diet. So what are the best ways to make a start?

• Eat at regular times to help your digestive system establish a routine.
• Eat little and often. Eating too much in one go can cause bloating and diarrhoea.

- Eat slowly. Gulping food quickly can cause you to swallow air, which results in wind and bloating.
- Chew your food well to give enzymes in your saliva more time to digest food and stimulate gastric juices.
- Drink plenty of fluids, especially water. Water combines with fibre in the intestine to make your stools bulkier and easier to pass and it rehydrates you if you have diarrhoea.
- Forget fatty foods. A balanced diet that focuses on plain foods and is low in saturated fats and sugar and highly spiced foods is likely to be of benefit. Fatty foods can trigger IBS because fat stimulates the liver to release bile to break it down. Bile contains acids that can irritate a sensitive gut. Foods that can cause this kind of problem include fried foods, full-fat dairy foods, fatty meats and chocolate.

4

Which diet?

The irritable bowel syndrome is a common and poorly understood chronic condition that is treated with a great variety of
drugs and other therapies without enduring success.

(Klein 1988)

You may be one of the lucky ones. You leave your doctor's surgery
clutching a prescription for an antispasmodic (to help the pain) plus
a bulk laxative (for constipation) plus, possibly, a short-term mild
antidepressant (to reduce stress), and they may work well and greatly
improve your IBS.

Or they may not. In the present state of medical knowledge, not
only is there no single definitive test which your doctor can use and
say, 'This test is positive, therefore you have irritable bowel syndrome',
there is also no single therapy that is reliably effective in the general
treatment of IBS. Until there is you will have to make do with whatever conventional or alternative medicine can offer, or with the vari-
ous things you can do to help yourself.

Although there is a lot you can do for yourself, never rush straight
into self-treatment, as you could overlook something serious. Visit
your doctor and get it properly diagnosed. (*Coping Successfully with
your Irritable Bowel* lists the guidelines for diagnosis, and will give you
confidence in your doctor's decision.) Conscientiously take whatever
he or she prescribes, and follow any advice you are given. Do whatever you can to reduce the stress in your life and, if necessary, make
changes to your diet.

Unfortunately, there is also no one special diet to make the irritable
bowel less irritable. Until quite recently bran was the standard recommended treatment, but that is probably not as effective as was origi-
nally thought, and some people find it makes their condition worse.
Many people with digestive troubles increase the amount of fibre in
their diet, including brown bread and grains. However, while these
foods don't cause IBS, they can make it worse in up to 55 per cent of
those who have it, research shows, so that it may be worth easing up

on high-fibre foods. Some experts (such as Professor Peter Whorwell of Manchester University) suggest avoiding all cereal grains (wheat, oats and other grains) for three months to see if it makes a difference. This is part of dietary treatment for many people with IBS. See Appendix 3, page 79 for further details of the low-fibre diet recommended by Addenbrooke's Hospital in Cambridge. Where a particular food is the cause of the problem the diet will have to be specially modified.

So what should you do?

First, think carefully about your symptoms and follow the advice given in my earlier book. Then consider how you can adapt your diet. A high-fibre diet will usually help constipation, a low-fibre diet often helps diarrhoea and wind, and individual problem foods can be identified with an exclusion diet.

Constipation or diarrhoea

Before deciding whether constipation or diarrhoea is your main symptom, it is as well to be aware of exactly what these conditions really are. Do you have several bowel movements every day? If so, is this really diarrhoea? Or do you have one every few days, and if so, is this constipation?

True diarrhoea is the passing of unformed watery stools, whether this happens frequently or not. True constipation is passing small hard stools and often involves straining to do so. 'Pseudo-diarrhoea' may be described as having frequent bowel movements that are not unformed and watery, and may even be hard and pelletty, and 'pseudo-constipation' as having to strain to pass normally formed or even loose stools (types 4, 5, 6 or 7 on the scale below). With pseudo-constipation you may also experience a feeling of incomplete evacuation – the sensation after a bowel movement that there is more to come. Dr K.W. Heaton and his colleagues at Bristol Royal Infirmary did some very interesting work on these two conditions, and produced a simple method of helping their patients to decide whether they have diarrhoea or constipation. They devised the Bristol stool form scale, or Meyers scale as it is sometimes called, and I am grateful to Dr Heaton for permission to reproduce it here.

Over the next few days, look carefully at the stools you produce (if you have read my previous book this should not embarrass you at all!) and see which description fits best. These days, you can even buy Bristol stool scale merchandise in the form of a pack of cards, a puzzle, a hand towel or a gift mug!

The Bristol stool form scale shows:

1 Separate hard lumps like nuts
2 Sausage-shaped but lumpy
3 Like a sausage or snake but with cracks on its surface
4 Like a sausage or snake, smooth and soft
5 Soft blobs with clear-cut edges
6 Fluffy pieces with ragged edges, a mushy stool
7 Watery, no solid pieces.

If your stools fit numbers 1 and 2, and to a much lesser extent number 3, this is constipation even if you have a bowel movement like this several times a day. So you should avoid anything that is likely to make you more constipated, eat a diet high in dietary fibre, and ask your doctor whether bulking agents such as Fybogel, Isogel or lactulose would be helpful to make your bowel movement softer and more bulky; they are available on prescription and over the counter. Linseeds are often recommended as a non-inflammatory source of Omega 3 which may help soothe the over-sensitive gut and prevent it from over-reacting. They are sometimes also recommended for bloating. The British Dietetic Association recommends that if your symptoms involve constipation you try adding one tablespoon a day of brown or golden linseeds to breakfast cereal, yogurt, soup or salad. Have a small glass of fluid with each tablespoon of linseeds. You may have them whole or ground, though some people find them more effective when freshly ground; another option is to soak them overnight in yogurt or a probiotic milk product, when they become much softer and more chewy. Bran (wheat bran, soya bran or rice bran) may be helpful if you have abdominal pain plus constipation, but possibly not as effective as bulking agents, and not as palatable; oats might be a better choice instead. For example, you could try porridge with a little linseed sprinkled on top. If one type (bran, for example) has not improved your symptoms after three months, try another type (such as a bulking agent), as people differ in their responses to different types of fibre. Drink several pints of fluid a day while on a high-fibre diet.

Keep on the high-fibre diet for a few weeks, but if it appears to make your IBS worse change to a low-fibre diet for about a month (see Appendix 3, page 79). While you are on a low-fibre diet it is important to take bulking agents such as Fybogel, Isogel or lactulose to prevent constipation. If neither high-fibre nor low-fibre diets appear to work, try an exclusion diet to see if you have an intolerance to any particular food (see page 26).

Number 4 on the scale is a normal healthy bowel movement. If your stools are soft, bulky and easy to pass you should not be having serious problems. If you are, discuss it with your doctor. If your stools fit the description of numbers 6 and 7 this is diarrhoea, even if you have only one bowel movement a day.

A high-fibre diet (especially if you take bran) will probably not do much good if your stools are already normal or loose (types 4, 5, 6 or 7) and may even make things worse. So try a low-fibre diet (see Appendix 3, page 79) to give your gut a rest for a few weeks, especially if the problem started after a bout of holiday diarrhoea. While on the low-fibre diet, it is important to keep taking Fybogel, Isogel or lactulose to prevent constipation. If a low-fibre diet doesn't work, it may be that you have a food intolerance, in which case two weeks on an exclusion diet (see page 26) should help identify this. If an exclusion diet brings no relief, then it is highly likely that your IBS is not caused or triggered by problem foods, and you should look for some other cause, such as stress.

5

Making a start

The high-fibre diet has been the traditional first-line approach to irritable bowel syndrome. It therefore seems a good way to start. If simple constipation is your main IBS symptom a diet like this will probably be effective, and it should reduce abdominal pain too.

High-fibre diet

Eat plenty of:

- wholemeal bread
- wholemeal flour
- brown rice
- high-fibre breakfast cereals like All-Bran
- potatoes in their jackets
- green leafy vegetables like spinach, broccoli and leeks.

Other good sources of fibre are:

- baked beans (though they may cause uncomfortable 'wind')
- spring greens
- brussels sprouts
- cabbage
- carrots
- beans – broad, butter, runner, French, red kidney
- lentils
- sweetcorn (some people find this makes their IBS worse)
- frozen peas
- apples
- apricots
- bananas
- raspberries
- avocados
- figs

- dates
- blackberries
- prunes (stewed)
- blackcurrants
- redcurrants
- gooseberries
- rhubarb (some people find this makes their IBS worse).

As mentioned before, it is important to drink plenty of fluids to ensure the fibre works well without drawing fluid from elsewhere in your body. If you are worried about your weight, keep to low-calorie fluids, such as skimmed milk (which keeps up your intake of calcium), water and herb tea. Low-calorie canned drinks may contain additives which upset your intestines.

Bran works well for many people, although some find it makes things worse. It reduces pressure in the large intestine, speeds up the passage of food through the digestive system and absorbs water, thus making the stools softer, bulkier and easier to pass. Take 1 tablespoon two or three times a day with meals, but be prepared to increase or decrease this amount according to the reaction you get; you will need to take less if you get abdominal pain and a bloated uncomfortable feeling, and to take more if it doesn't appear to work. Stick with it for several weeks, as it can take up to three months to see how well it works.

Low-fibre diet

Did the high-fibre diet make your IBS worse? Is diarrhoea your main symptom? Or has an attack of holiday diarrhoea started it off again? If so, you might benefit from a low-fibre diet.

The Gastroenterology Research Department of Addenbrooke's Hospital, Cambridge, recommend a low-fibre diet to some of their IBS patients, and I am grateful to Professor John Hunter for permission to reproduce it here, with the patient information sheet, in Appendix 3 (p. 79); you can check for updates to this at <www.cambridgeshire. nhs.uk/SHP%20downloads/Workstreams/Gastro/Low%20fibre%20 diet%20sheet.pdf>.

Because a low-fibre diet contains very little dietary fibre (roughage) it is important to use a bulk laxative such as Isogel, Fybogel or Normacol to keep preventing constipation.

Let us now suppose that the high-fibre diet has not worked, and nor has the low-fibre one. What next?

Exclusion diet

This is probably the time to consider whether you might have an intolerance to a particular food (or foods). Food intolerance is a more likely possibility if diarrhoea is your main IBS problem, and also if you have any allergic condition such as asthma, some forms of eczema, hay fever, rhinitis or urticaria.

Obviously the first step is to conscientiously remove from your diet those foods that you know for certain disagree with you. Don't touch them for two weeks, and see whether your symptoms improve during this time. For many people this in itself will be enough. Then introduce the culprit food in an average-size helping just to check whether it is indeed the villain; if you get no unpleasant reaction you will at least know you can eat that food. If your symptoms return, cut that food out of your diet for up to six months before trying again. You may find that after giving your intestines a rest from it you can take it occasionally in small quantities without too much ill-effect.

However, it may be that you are really quite uncertain which foods are triggering your IBS, in which case a more systematic approach is needed.

Because there is no conclusive medical test for food intolerance, the 'test' most commonly used to pinpoint problem foods is an exclusion diet. In its harshest form, patients existed on nothing but lamb, pears and mineral water for one to two weeks, and then gradually introduced new foods, noting which foods caused an adverse reaction. Fortunately, exclusion diets such as that one would only be used in the most extreme circumstance, with the patient in hospital under the close direction of a gastroenterologist and dietitian.

Many gastroenterologists, general practitioners and dietitians have devised their own exclusion diets as a means of finding which foods disagree with individual patients. The one that is used here has been developed by the Gastroenterology Research Department of Addenbrooke's Hospital, Cambridge, and I am grateful to Dr John Hunter for permission to reprint it here. It allows you to eat a wide range of foods to give a healthy balanced diet, it has been very well tested, and when used under the direction of a competent clinician it can resolve symptoms in about 50 per cent of patients.

If you have any doubts about your general state of health you should ask your general practitioner whether it would be a good idea for you to try an exclusion diet. Or arrange to see a qualified dietitian for advice. Be wary of undertaking any major change to your diet unsupervised, and don't use an exclusion diet on children except under medical supervision. If you have not had your IBS diagnosed by a doctor, this might be a good time to do it, to make sure you are not overlooking a more serious condition; in any case, you need to be sure you are treating the right thing.

You can read more about this exclusion diet in a wide range of books – see 'References and further reading'.

The foods you can and can't eat are listed in Table 5.1. You can eat anything in the 'allowed' column, and nothing in the 'not allowed' column. *It is important to keep strictly to the diet for two weeks.* It won't work if it is done half-heartedly. Having one of the forbidden foods even once could make it almost impossible to work out which foods disagree with you. But by taking time and commitment to do it

Table 5.1 Exclusion diet

	Not allowed	Allowed
Meat	Beef, sausages Beefburgers Meat pies	All other meats Poultry and game Ham and bacon
Fish	Fish in batter or breadcrumbs	White fish, fatty fish Smoked fish, tinned tuna in brine Tinned sardines in soya oil Prawns
Vegetables	Potatoes Onions Sweetcorn Tinned vegetables in sauce	All other fresh vegetables Salad Pulses – beans, peas, lentils Tinned vegetables, such as tomatoes Tomato puree
Fruit	Citrus fruit, e.g. oranges, satsumas, grapefruit, lemons	All other fruit – fresh or tinned – e.g. apples, pears, pineapple
Cereals	Wheat, e.g. bread, cakes, biscuits, pasta, noodles, semolina Breakfast cereals, e.g. Weetabix, Shredded Wheat Rye, e.g. Ryvita	Rice Ground rice, rice flour Rice Krispies, puffed rice cereal Rice cakes Arrowroot Tapioca

	Oats	Sago
	Barley	Millet
	Corn, e.g. cornflakes,	Buckwheat
	cornflour, custard powder	

Cooking oils	Corn oil	Sunflower oil
	Vegetable oil	Safflower oil
		Soya oil,
		Olive oil

Dairy	Cow's milk – all types	Soya milk
products	Dried milk	Soya yogurt, soya ice cream
	Tinned milk	Tofu
	Goat's milk	Milk-free margarine
	Butter	Tomor, Vitasieg
	Cream	Granose – vegetable margarine
	Margarine	Pure, Suma
	Yogurt	
	Cheese	
	Eggs	

Beverages	Tea	Herbal teas, e.g. redbush,
	Coffee	rosehip, camomile
	Decaffeinated tea and coffee	Fresh fruit juices, e.g. apple,
	Fruit squashes	pineapple, tomato, grape juice
	Canned drinks	Ribena
	Orange juice	Mineral water, e.g. Evian,
	Grapefruit juice	Scottish Highland, etc.
	Lemon juice	
	Alcohol	
	Tap water – discuss with	
	the dietician	

Miscellaneous	Marmalade, jams	Pure fruit spread
	containing preservatives	Homemade jam
	and colours	Salt, herbs, black pepper
	Mustard	Spices in moderation
	Yeast	Sugar, honey
	Yeast extract, e.g. Marmite	Brown rice miso
	Gravy mixes	Gravy browning containing
	Vinegar	caramel and salt only
	Nuts	Dried fruit (wash first)
	Baking powder	Dried banana, coconut,
	containing wheat	sunflower seeds
	Chocolate	Baking powder – gluten-free
		or Sainsbury's
		Carob

properly there's a better than evens chance you will improve your IBS beyond all recognition.

The list of foods in the 'not allowed' column may seem rather daunting at first, but there is such a good range of foods in the 'allowed' column that you shouldn't have much difficulty following this diet for two weeks. But in case you feel there is nothing left to eat, here is a list of possible meals for one week (individual recipes are given at the end of this chapter for dishes marked with an asterisk in order to avoid wheat or dairy products).

Two-week exclusion diet

This diet excludes all those foods which are most likely to cause food intolerance. The diet must be followed for two weeks. Recipes for dishes marked * are on pages 33–4.

Keep a diary during this period recording food eaten and symptoms.

Breakfast

- Home-made muesli*
- Stewed fruit (apples, apricots, prunes) with or without goat's milk or yogurt, and sweetened with honey
- Rice crackers, with non-dairy spread and jam or honey
- Rice Krispies (or any cereal that does not contain wheat, corn, oats or rye – check packet labels carefully), with a milk substitute or fruit juice
- Apple, pineapple or tomato juice
- Herb tea.

Day 1	lunch:	cauliflower in cheese sauce*; raw apple
	supper:	avocado salad, with apple and beetroot in yogurt dressing*; banana jelly*
Day 2	lunch:	buckwheat croquettes* with vegetables; melon
	supper:	grilled trout with mushrooms and peas; baked pears with honey
Day 3	lunch:	home-made soup*; bananas
	supper:	grilled lamb's liver, mushrooms, carrots, cauliflower; baked apple stuffed with sultanas and honey
Day 4	lunch:	green pepper stuffed with rice and mushrooms; mixed dried fruit soaked overnight in apple juice
	supper:	leeks/cauliflower/celery/courgettes/green beans (according to season) in cheese sauce*; fresh fruit (not citrus)

Day 5   lunch: lentil rissoles (taste better if made the day before);
                     fresh fruit (not citrus)
           supper: grilled lamb chops and vegetables (not potatoes,
                     onions, cabbage or sweetcorn); rice pudding*
Day 6   lunch: grilled chicken (hot or cold) with salad of apple,
                     courgette, cauliflower or cucumber; stewed fruit
           supper: stir-fry of sprouting vegetables with any other
                     vegetables except potatoes, cabbage, onions or
                     sweetcorn, and flavoured with tamari (a wheat-
                     free soya sauce); baked bananas (cooked with
                     honey and non-dairy margarine)
Day 7   lunch: grilled white fish with vegetables; fresh fruit (not
                     citrus)
           supper: risotto with creamed spinach*, leftover chicken
                     and any other vegetables; fresh fruit salad (with
                     no citrus fruits).

With any luck you will now feel that spending two weeks on an exclusion diet is not impossible, and that you can eat varied interesting meals.

However, be prepared that the first few days on the exclusion diet
may be unpleasant as your body gets used to being without the foods
it has had regularly. This is usually a *good* sign. You should feel much
better in about a week, so stick with the diet, and don't be tempted to
give up if you feel worse at the very beginning. If you continue to feel
worse after about a week, it could be that a new replacement food is
the culprit, especially if you are eating a lot of it to substitute for a food
in the 'not allowed' column; if this happens, you will need to cut out
any new food that you have introduced.

In addition to the foods in the 'not allowed' column, exclude any
foods that you know disagree with you. With any luck you will only
have to go without them for the two weeks you are on the diet, and
there are lots of acceptable alternatives (see Appendix 2).

Eat as wide a variety as possible from the foods in the 'allowed'
column, to ensure a healthy balanced diet. Keep an accurate diary of
everything you eat, as well as any symptoms you have and when they
occur. Any symptoms you notice will probably have been caused by
one of the foods eaten in the previous 24 hours, and this should help
you pinpoint the source of the trouble.

You should see a steady improvement in your IBS symptoms during
the second week, and if this happens you can gradually start to re-
introduce new foods, in the following order:

1 Tap water
2 Potatoes
3 Cow's milk
4 Yeast
5 Tea
6 Rye
7 Butter
8 Onions
9 Eggs
10 Oats
11 Coffee
12 Chocolate
13 Barley
14 Citrus fruits
15 Corn
16 Cow's cheese
17 White wine
18 Shellfish
19 Cow's yogurt
20 Vinegar
21 Wheat
22 Nuts
23 Preservatives
24 Processed foods.

Introduce these new foods at the rate of one every two days; eat a good-sized portion of it, not just a tiny nibble. During this time continue to keep your diary of everything you eat, the symptoms you get and when. Only by doing this will you know which newly introduced food is the cause of your symptoms. If you have a bad reaction to something, flush out your digestive system by drinking plenty of water; adding a little bicarbonate of soda helps.

When you have reintroduced all the foods, go back and test them again to be sure. If only one or two less common foods are the culprit, this should be no problem, as there are acceptable substitutes for almost everything. But if you now find that many foods trigger your symptoms, and especially if basic foods like wheat and dairy products are among them, arrange to see a dietitian to make sure the diet you must follow in future will be nutritionally adequate.

Having found which foods disagree with you, keep off them for about six months, to give your digestive system a complete rest from them. Then try again after another six months, and so on. If the time comes when that food causes no reaction, eat it once a week to begin with, then perhaps twice a week, but never every day. You will have to be your own judge about how often you can eat it.

If after two weeks on the exclusion diet you are not feeling considerably better, food intolerance is probably *not* the cause of your IBS symptoms. In this case see if your doctor has any other treatment to offer, or consider some form of alternative therapy such as osteopathy, homoeopathy, acupuncture, medical herbalism or hypnotherapy (see the box below).

If you get a lot of pain after meals, try a low-fat diet; but don't cut out fats altogether, as they are important for the correct working of the body. Choose foods marked 'low-fat' and select lean cuts of meat, low-fat meats such as chicken, turkey and rabbit; avoid higher-fat fish such as mackerel and herring.

Gut-centred hypnotherapy

Gut-centred hypnotherapy has shown good results in people with IBS, giving them more control over their condition and achieving positive results in 70 per cent of patients. As well as reducing sensitivity and contractions in the gut itself, hypnotherapy also eases other symptoms such as tiredness and gynaecological pain. Gut-centred hypnotherapy was pioneered by Professor Peter Whorwell, professor of medicine and gastroenterology at the University of Manchester and director of the South Manchester Functional Bowel Service, a leading centre for IBS treatment. Professor Whorwell also led the development group that put together the first guidelines on IBS for doctors.

European studies also back up the effectiveness of hypnotherapy. Research from the University of Gothenburg, Sweden, and a previous study published in the *Scandinavian Journal of Gastroenterology* found that not only did hypnotherapy help alleviate IBS discomfort but the effects were long-term – up to seven years.

In gut-centred hypnotherapy, people visualise the gut as a smooth-flowing river. The aim is to make the river flow smoothly, without blockages (such as constipation or wind) or flooding (such as diarrhoea). So, for example, constipation might be visualised as rocks which are blocking the river and have to be removed, while diarrhoea might be imaged as a fast-flowing river, to be slowed down or partially dammed by bulwarks, wider banks or extra sand.

Hypnotherapy empowers those with IBS by helping them control their symptoms through deep relaxation and individually attuned hypnotic suggestion. Relieving anxiety helps the gut become more relaxed and less sensitive, so reducing symptoms. It's also thought that hypnotherapy may have an impact on the part of the brain involved in processing pain, the anterior cingulate cortex (ACC). It is thought that hypnotherapy may reduce activity in the ACC, so again reducing people's perception of gut discomfort.

Recipes for dishes marked *

Muesli

Mix together buckwheat (no relation to wheat, despite its name) or millet with dried fruits such as apricots, raisins, sultanas and chopped apple. Serve with a milk substitute (such as soya milk) and honey. Some other recipes for wheat-free muesli are on page 42.

Cheese sauce

Melt 25 g (1 oz) non-dairy margarine, blend in 25 g (1 oz) soya flour, cook for about 1 minute, then slowly mix in 250 ml (10 fl oz) soya milk, stirring all the time with a wooden spoon. When thoroughly blended add 50–75 g (2–3 oz) non-dairy cheese (or any other flavouring that you prefer) and stir until melted.

Yogurt dressing

Mix goat's milk yogurt with chopped mint, chives, garlic and seasoning (unless you know any of these disagree with you).

Banana jelly

Sprinkle a sachet of gelatine on 100 ml (3 fl oz) of heated apple juice and stir until dissolved. Make up to 500 ml (1 pint) with more apple juice. Add sliced bananas. Leave to set. (Other fruits can be used to give variety.)

Buckwheat croquettes

Cook 150 g (6 oz) buckwheat in twice its own volume of water until the water has been absorbed and the buckwheat is soft; drain and cool. Add finely chopped celery/carrots/leeks, 25 g (1 oz) soya flour, seasoning and herbs. Shape into rounds 1.25 cm (½ inch) thick, and fry on both sides until cooked.

Soup

Cook together plenty of suitable chopped or shredded vegetables, and a cup of red lentils, without salt until soft. Mix them all in a blender. Add seasoning and water until the liquid has a soup-like consistency. If you have a microwave or pressure cooker, soup like this can be made very quickly. See Chapter 7 for soup recipes.

Rice pudding

Sprinkle 75 g (3 oz) flaked rice onto 500 ml (1 pint) of near-boiling milk-substitute. Simmer for 10–15 minutes (or according to directions on packet). Sweeten with honey, and serve alone or with stewed fruit.

Creamed spinach

Cook spinach in a very small quantity of water without salt until it can be easily chopped into a pulp. Add non-dairy margarine, and seasoning, and mix together until creamy.

6

Putting your diet into practice

Hopefully by now you have a good idea of what you should or should not be eating. Whether your problem is mainly constipation or mainly diarrhoea, whether you need a high-fibre or a low-fibre diet, and whether there are certain foods you know make your IBS worse, you should still try to eat a diet that is healthy, balanced, varied and acceptable to you.

Even if you have to be careful about what you eat, there is no need to feel 'different'. Many people find they have to be careful about something or other – it's quite normal. Once you get used to what you can and can't eat you will find you adapt to it quite quickly, and it shouldn't greatly affect your life.

The important thing is to eat a healthy diet, whatever your age, and to eat calmly. It is surprising how many young people develop IBS when they leave home. No more sitting round the family table eating in a quiet leisurely way a meal that Mother has prepared; once young people are out in the big world their lives become more stressful, and many of them eat 'on the hoof', making do with junk food that requires little or no preparation, and doing it all in a hurry.

Even not-so-young men and women with IBS tend to be much the same: a rushed breakfast (or none at all), lunch eaten perched on a bar stool, or dashing between A and B, and ending with a rich supper washed down with too much alcohol – the perfect environment for irritable bowel syndrome!

Mothers of young children also tend to rush around at mealtimes – leaping up and down between the table and the cooker, attending to children, grabbing a sandwich with one hand while mopping up spills with the other, and generally putting their own needs last. Make a point of sitting down at mealtimes with your children, making their eating enjoyable as well as your own.

If you have IBS, it is quite likely that at least part of your life is tense and stressful. Yet it is important to be emotionally relaxed when eating, or else your IBS gets worse. Try to follow the following rules:

- Don't eat when you are tense, upset, angry or anxious.
- Allow plenty of time for each meal.
- Don't eat standing up or 'on the hoof' or perched on a stool – sit down on a chair.
- 'Grazing' (eating as you move about) may be fashionable, but it does the digestive system no good at all.
- Take time to shop for, and prepare, wholesome foods.
- Try not to swallow air when you are eating.
- Decide in advance how much you are going to eat, and don't be tempted to eat more.
- Stop eating as soon as you feel full.
- Cut down on rich food.
- Try to leave two to three hours between your last meal and going to bed.

Think carefully before you embark on a crash diet. Many women can trace their IBS back to such a diet, possibly triggered by a sudden drop in fibre and taking a different range of foods. Crash dieting can induce constipation, which in itself can cause IBS symptoms and may then be followed by diarrhoea.

There are now well-recognised guidelines for healthy eating, so try to follow them. For example:

- Trim excess fat off meat before cooking.
- Grill rather than fry.
- Avoid deep-fat frying.
- Use fresh fruit and vegetables rather than tinned or frozen or processed.
- Eat the skins of boiled or baked potatoes.
- Use as little salt as possible in cooking and at table.
- Eat brown bread, pasta and rice in preference to white.
- Have some leafy green vegetables every day.
- Substitute fresh food for processed food wherever possible.

Simply following these guidelines could work wonders for your IBS, especially if you are bothered by constipation and abdominal pain; but it is also important to eat in a calm relaxed way, giving your digestive system the opportunity to work properly.

Give time, too, to choosing what you eat. If you don't think about this in advance, you will probably find it is time for the next meal and you haven't got anything to eat; so you rush to the nearest shop and choose something that you can cook and eat in no time at all – and then wonder why you have stomach ache. It is a good idea to sit down quietly for about 20 minutes a week, and write down on paper what you will have for each meal. Perhaps you will choose some of the recipes in Chapter 7, or from any book on good healthy eating, or from one of the many internet recipe sites. When you have decided what you will have for each meal, make out a shopping list and buy everything all at once – that way you will always have something good and nutritious in the house, and won't be tempted to eat junk food because you are in a hurry.

No matter what you are cutting out from your diet, you should have no difficulty finding acceptable alternatives. Here are some ideas for creative eating on a restricted diet:

- Legumes (lentils, beans, etc.) are a useful low-cost, high-protein alternative to meat, and can be made into numerous delicious meals. Get into the habit of putting some on to soak in a bowl or saucepan at bedtime or before you go to work, so they are ready to cook when you need them.
- Rice cakes are a good alternative to bread and biscuits if you can't take wheat.
- You can make your own rice flour by grinding rice very finely, but it cooks rather differently from wheat flour, so experiment first.
- Have you tried tofu? Gram for gram it is the cheapest and richest source of protein available except for eggs. Tofu is made from soyabean, is low in salt and saturated fat and is free from cholesterol. Although almost tasteless in itself, it absorbs the flavours of other ingredients. It is available in most health food shops and many supermarkets, and is highly nutritious – and also an ideal slimming food. Handle tofu gently; when you get it home, unwrap it and put it in the fridge in a bowl of water, completely covered so it doesn't absorb other flavours. Change the water daily. It will keep fresh for about a week from the day it was made.
- Nowadays we expect foods to keep for weeks or even months, but this is usually only possible by adding preservatives and other additives which may make your IBS worse, so be prepared to accept more natural storage times.

Other substitutes are:
- *Drinks*: herb teas, grape juice, apple juice, blackcurrant juice, pineapple juice, tomato juice, vegetable juice

- *Quick snacks*: sunflower seeds, sesame seed bars
- *Spreads*: jams containing only sugar, fruit and pectin; honey
- *Cooking oils*: corn oil, sunflower oil, safflower oil – all slightly more expensive than ordinary salad or vegetable oils, but much better for you
- *Flavourings*: cinnamon, nutmeg, parsley, paprika, celery salt, pepper, vanilla, carob
- *Tap water*: bottled spring water is an obvious substitute, but if you find tap water disagrees with you, you should see your doctor before eliminating it.

As mentioned earlier, don't cut out staple foods from your diet without talking to your doctor or a qualified dietitian. To find a state registered dietitian, try your doctor's receptionist, or the dietetics department of your local hospital, or write to the British Dietetic Association (see 'Useful addresses').

If you are eating a restricted diet, you may be considering taking dietary supplements (vitamin pills, etc.) to make up for the short-fall in your diet. As a general rule, these should not be necessary – most people who eat a balanced diet have little or no need of them. However, if you eat no wheat products you may become deficient in B-group vitamins, and if you eat no dairy products you will need to get enough calcium from somewhere, so for you supplements may be the answer. If in doubt, ask your doctor.

Some supplements have been found to be helpful for people with IBS:

- Mint: the *British Medical Journal* reported in 2008 that nearly 50 per cent of IBS sufferers found relief from their symptoms when they took peppermint oil. Try a few drops of peppermint oil in hot water, or you can take peppermint tea, or try it in herb or capsule form.
- Calcium: as calcium slows down gut contractions, a calcium supplement may help to counteract diarrhoea.
- Rice water: for episodes of acute diarrhoea, take the water in which rice has been boiled, with a little salt or a pinch of organic stock. It's surprisingly delicious – and can be effective!
- Probiotics: research has shown that probiotics can reduce bloating and ease constipation in IBS, thanks to their ability to alter gut flora and boost immunity. Why not try a probiotic yogurt, fermented milk drink or supplement to see if it improves symptoms? Take daily for at least four weeks. And maybe try another brand if they don't appear to be helping.

- Turmeric: studies suggest that turmeric can ease digestive problems, owing to its anti-inflammatory properties and its ability to block abnormal muscle contractions in the gut. The recommended dosage is 500 mg of turmeric extract once a day until symptoms improve.

Unfortunately, many people who live life in the fast lane feel that it is enough to eat a totally inadequate diet and then compensate by taking vitamins, minerals and other supplements in the form of pills, potions and powders. Many use dietary supplements as a substitute for sensible living. Instead of reducing the stress in their lives they take 'stress-reducing pills'; instead of tackling the causes of insomnia they take sleeping pills; instead of eating plenty of roughage and worrying less about minor constipation they take laxatives. Your IBS may well have been caused by the life you lead, and it is not possible to prevent or reverse the ravages of a bad lifestyle with a pill. Nutrition by pills is not nutrition; we should not deceive ourselves that it is.

7

Ideas and recipes for healthy living

As mentioned before, one of the main things your irritable bowel needs is good healthy food eaten in a calm leisurely way. Anything else is asking for trouble. Whether you are a stressed business man or woman, a harassed parent or a working person in a hurry, time spent planning, cooking and eating wholesome sensible food will be a worthwhile investment. The alternative is all the awful symptoms of irritable bowel syndrome.

'Wholesome sensible food' is not the kiss of death. You can forget all about boiled fish, gruel, sheep's head broth, calves' foot jelly, dumplings with barley, groats, breadcrumbs with dripping, bread-and-milk, sago and tapioca. Just flicking through the recipes that follow should convince you that eating to please your irritable bowel can be quick, interesting and cheap.

Many of the recipes in this chapter are wheat-free, as this is a harder diet to follow. Look out for WF to indicate wheat-free recipes. However, the majority of people with IBS should be thinking less about a wheat-free diet and more about a high-fibre diet, so unless you know that you must avoid wheat you should be using wholemeal bread and wholemeal flour rather than wheat-free bread and flour. There are many high-fibre diet cookbooks around – your local library or bookshops will probably have several, as will internet booksellers, and the internet is a rich source of recipes.

If wheat disagrees with you, you can choose to eat it just occasionally or in very small quantities (see Chapter 3 on food intolerance) in the hope that your gut can cope with it, or use a recipe with a wheat-free flour such as Doves Farm or Glutafin (see 'Useful addresses' for stockists).

If dairy products disagree with you, you can choose to eat them occasionally or in very small quantities, as with wheat. Or you can use substitute products such as soya milk instead of cow's or goat's milk, and non-dairy spreads instead of ordinary butter and margarine, according to how your digestive system reacts to dairy products.

If you have problems with other foods (such as onions, citrus fruits, chocolate or potato, for example) you should check each recipe carefully, and either leave out the offending food or choose a different recipe. Equally, some recipes include pre-prepared ingredients, such as stock cubes, for convenience. Do check that they don't contain any E numbers that give you problems.

Breakfast

Do you grab a cup of coffee some time between getting up and starting the day, and call this 'breakfast'? Do you perch at the breakfast bar, drinking coffee with one hand and shaving or putting on make-up with the other? Do you get up about five minutes before you have to leave for work? Are you in such a rush to get the children off to school that you don't have any time to sit down and relax? If so, then it's hardly surprising you have irritable bowel syndrome!

It really needn't be like this. As you will have read in *Coping Successfully with your Irritable Bowel*, it is important to allow plenty of time at the start of the day for a relaxed breakfast and then to disappear to the toilet for ten minutes or more to make sure you do not get constipated. The 'bowel-emptying' message is strongest after meals, and particularly first thing in the morning, and you ignore it at your peril. It is highly likely that your irritable bowel is caused by the life you lead, so the start of a new day is a good time to begin a different way of doing things.

So, get up early enough to allow yourself plenty of time in the morning. Always eat breakfast, sitting down at the table in a quiet leisurely way; reading a morning paper or magazine is a good way to prolong breakfast. If coffee disagrees with you, drink tea, herb tea, Barleycup, Caro or other alternatives; you'll quickly get used to them. Remember that many people with IBS drink far more coffee than is good for them, and if your digestive system is more sensitive than other people's, you don't want to be aggravating it unnecessarily.

If citrus fruits disagree with you, try apple juice, tomato juice, pineapple juice, etc.

Provided you are not sensitive to wheat or on a low-fibre diet, eat a high-fibre cereal, followed by wholemeal toast; and perhaps some stewed fruit like apricots or prunes.

If wheat is a problem, you could try one of the following.

Stewed fruit

Put some dried fruit (apricots, prunes, mixed dried fruit, for example) in a bowl covered with plenty of water (or cold tea) and leave to soak for several hours until soft. You can speed the process up by bringing the water gently to the boil first. Add sugar as necessary. Serve hot or cold.

Eggs

These can be boiled, poached, baked or scrambled.

Muesli

The following are three recipes for non-wheat muesli – you can add or take away ingredients according to taste.

Mix together combinations of dry ingredients, and keep in a food storage jar. At bedtime put some of the dry mixture in a cereal bowl, cover with water or apple juice, and leave to soak overnight. At breakfast serve with fresh fruit or dried fruit or yogurt.

6 tablespoons flaked millet	4 tablespoons flaked rice WF
2 tablespoons chopped nuts	1 teaspoon chopped dried fruit
1 teaspoon toasted sesame seeds	

4 tablespoons flaked rice	4 tablespoons oatmeal WF
1 tablespoon sunflower seeds	1 tablespoon chopped nuts
1 tablespoon raisins, sultanas or currants	

4 tablespoons of any of the following (or a mixture): medium oatmeal, rolled oats, barley flakes, millet flakes, rye flakes, with 1 tablespoon of soya or rice bran.   WF

You can also add to any muesli: sesame seeds, sunflower seeds, any dried fruit (such as dates, apricots, raisins, sultanas, peaches), any nuts (walnuts, hazelnuts, almonds, cashews, brazils, etc.) and any fresh fruit that doesn't disagree with you.

It is worth visiting a wholefood or health food shop to buy the basic ingredients once every week or two, and spending a few minutes mixing them together. Experiment first with small quantities until you find the combination you like, then make up a large quantity and keep it in a food storage jar.

Midday meal at work

How has your day gone so far? Did you get up in a rush? Miss breakfast? Dash out of the house, stand in an overcrowded train or bus, or sit in a traffic jam tapping your fingers impatiently on the steering wheel while you talked on your hands-free mobile or planned the day's work? Have you just finished the first of many cups of coffee while doing a hundred and one other things? Not a good start to the day!

And now it's somewhere between noon and 2 p.m., and time for something to eat. What will you have? A packet of crisps? A cigarette and a cup of coffee? A Pot Noodle? A chocolate bar? After all, you're so busy you haven't got any time to eat properly, have you? You have time to sit in traffic jams, work late, play squash or slump in front of the telly, but eating, shopping, cooking . . . ? No, of course not. And then you wonder why your gut plays you up!

Ultimately, of course, the choice is yours. As you will have read in my previous book, you can decide whether to continue with the very lifestyle that provokes your irritable bowel, or you can make a few changes here and there and, with luck, bring it under your control. Reducing stress is one important way; looking at how and what you eat is another.

The midday meal can be an obvious problem. You may have to eat a lot of business lunches, or spend your lunch hour rushing around doing the family shopping; you may feel you want to go out to the pub with your colleagues, or you may not like the food in the canteen. And if, on top of all this, certain foods disagree with you, any form of eating out can be stressful. Will the boeuf stroganoff have onions in it? Does the pizza have a wheat base? Will the sauce on the lasagne contain cow's milk? Can you have a ploughman's without cheese?

Consider, too, all the additives that are part and parcel of instant food: colourings, emulsifiers, stabilisers, thickeners, preservatives, antioxidants, flavour enhancers and flavourings. Very few restaurants, and even fewer pubs and canteens, make their food entirely from scratch; they nearly all use catering-quality foods in one form or another, which tend to be high in additives.

So if you can take to work a dish that is easy to shop for and simple to make, you can avoid these problems. It is obviously more trouble to do this, but if it eases your irritable bowel you may decide it is worth it.

This is not a chapter of recipes, just a collection of ideas to make it easy for you to eat wholesome food in the middle of the day. Many of them require having access to a microwave or conventional cooker in order to reheat them, but more and more firms and offices now have a microwave, and if yours doesn't perhaps you could persuade the boss that it would be a good investment. The cost would be comparatively small, it would take up very little space, and by encouraging its employees to eat nutritiously in the middle of the day the organisation is investing in their health, which is a financially (and morally) sound thing to do.

Even if you cannot use a cooker or microwave, you will still find plenty of ideas here for a quick, easy and nutritionally healthy midday meal.

- Invest in some suitable containers – a vacuum flask, a sandwich box, one or two plastic bowls with lids, some containers for reheating food in a microwave, or anything else you might need to take food to work and cook and eat it there.
- To save time in the morning, most snacks can be made the previous night, wrapped in cling film or put in a plastic container and kept in the fridge overnight. Salads can also be packed loosely in plastic bags.
- There is more to a packed lunch than a curled-up ham sandwich. Try filling a pitta bread or a French stick. Whatever you use, put in plenty of filling.
- To save yourself time and effort, make enough for two or three meals, and freeze what you don't use for another day.
- Or make a basic meal, then vary it slightly for the next two or three days.
- Eat plenty of fruit, fresh or dried.
- Try to plan a whole week's lunchtime menus – it's a lot less hassle than having to think about it each day. Also by buying enough for the whole week you avoid going short and having to fall back on junk food. You've got to think about it sometime, and one long 'think' is a lot easier than five short ones!
- Each week buy a few fillings for sandwiches or pitta bread, and rotate them in combination. You could try:

sardines	grated carrot
tuna	dried figs or apricots
cucumber	finely chopped celery
cold lean meat	mushrooms
watercress	tomatoes
eggs – hardboiled or scrambled	mashed cooked lentils
beansprouts	hummus
sliced apple	cottage cheese

sliced courgettes	grated cheese

. . . and anything else you like.

- Baked potatoes are cheap, filling and nutritious, and can easily be filled at home and taken to work, although you will need a microwave to heat them up. Possible fillings are:

baked beans	baked beans and grated cheese
cheese	egg with mayonnaise
ham	prawns
bacon	mushrooms
chicken	cucumber
turkey	yogurt
tuna	homemade coleslaw
sliced lettuce or cabbage	grated carrot
scrambled egg, tomato and onion	

. . . and anything else, including leftovers.

- If you can't eat wheat, take some rice cakes to work instead of bread or biscuits; or make your own bread, crispbreads, chapatis, etc., from recipes on pages 56–62.
- If you can tolerate just a little wheat, rye crispbreads may suit you.
- Buy an empty flan case (most supermarkets sell them), and fill it with any combinations of fillings you like, possibly bound together with a cheese sauce, and take a slice to work. Freeze the rest, or if you don't have a freezer fill the flan case with different fillings in two or three segments, and cut each segment when you need it. It will keep for three or four days in a fridge.
- It's very easy to make your own yogurt: put into a bowl 1 tablespoon of plain yogurt (it doesn't have to be 'live' yogurt, as long as it has no additives such as preservatives). Heat 500 ml (1 pint) milk to 50°C (125°F) and pour carefully onto the yogurt in the bowl. Stir very gently, cover with a plate, and leave in a warm place overnight. By morning it should have set, and have a thin layer of liquid on the top. Drain off the liquid. Now you can put some into a plastic bowl with a lid, and take it to work. Add anything you like, such as:

chopped dried apricots	honey
a tin of mandarin oranges, drained	finely chopped apple or pear
sultanas	chopped prunes
hazelnuts	mashed banana
raspberries.	

- Keep back a tablespoon of this yogurt as the starter for the next batch you make. You can also add it to main dishes, use it instead of cream or as the base of delicious drinks, or instead of oil in salad dressings. Store it in a fridge.
- Take to work one or more of the salads on pages 55–56.
- Pizza is quick and easy to make, and convenient to take to work. Some supermarkets sell plain pizza bases for you to add your own ingredients.
- Pancakes, too, make a good midday meal, and can be filled with anything you like. Basic recipes are on page 53. Savoury pancakes usually need to be heated.
- Hummus is high in protein, easy to make and can be used as part of a salad or as a basic filling in sandwiches or pitta bread. The recipe is:

225 g (8 oz) chick peas, soaked overnight and cooked (much more quickly in a pressure cooker) or a 400 g (14 oz) can, drained (keep the liquid from cooked or drained chick peas)
1 clove garlic, crushed   1 tablespoon tahini (sesame cream)
3 tablespoons sunflower oil   2 tablespoons lemon juice

Put drained chick peas in liquidiser or food processor with all the other ingredients, and blend until smooth. If necessary add some of the drained liquid until the hummus has the consistency of soft whipped cream. (Make it stiffer for filling sandwiches.)

- To cut down on coffee, keep some fruit juice at work, or some herb teabags. Also keep some herb teabags in your pocket or bag for when you are visiting.
- Take some fruit to work every day.
- Some suggestions for instant snacks are:

sunflower seeds   potato crisps without additives
pumpkin seeds   popping corn
sesame seed bars   dried fruit
cashew nuts   desiccated coconut
pistachio nuts

Having gone to the trouble of planning, buying and preparing your midday meal, don't destroy the benefit by bolting it down as you rush from A to B. Find a quiet place, sit down in a comfortable chair. Give yourself permission to take time off to digest your meal and eat in peace.

Soups

Homemade soups are easy to make and are ideal to take to work in a vacuum flask. They are nutritious, and soups containing vegetables are a good source of dietary fibre (roughage).

Even if you can't be bothered to make a meal some evenings, a bowl of homemade soup with a hunk of thick bread is filling, healthy and cheap. Sprinkle grated cheese on it, and have some fresh fruit to follow – what could be more wholesome and delicious!

It's not difficult to get into the habit of making soup regularly, and each batch will last two or three days if you keep it in the fridge; or you can freeze the rest for another day. If you have a cooker or microwave at work, take it with you cold; if not, heat it up before you leave home and keep it hot in a vacuum flask.

Some of the recipes in this chapter do not give specific quantities – it's up to you to choose how much of each vegetable you like; even where specific quantities are given as guidance you can usually be as flexible as you like, and vary them according to your taste and what is available. Also you can make the soup thick or thin according to how much water or stock you add; there's nothing to stop you making soups so thick you can eat them with a fork! If you have got a blender or food processor it is easier to make 'creamed' soups than having to force the ingredients through a sieve; and a microwave or pressure cooker will greatly reduce the cooking time if you are using vegetables that take longer to cook, like parsnips, potatoes and pulses. Conversely, many people find a slow-cooker useful as it is possible to set it going in the morning before you go to work, and return to find the delicious odours of a homemade meal wafting through the house. What better way to reduce any IBS-associated stress? There are many useful internet sites featuring slow-cooking (such as <www.channel4. com/4food/recipes/popular-dishes/slow-cooker> or <www.bbc.co.uk/ food/slow-cooked_dishes>). Even if you have none of these implements, you can still make delicious wholesome soups.

You can use any vegetables, and in any combination. If you cream the soup in a blender or food processor, adding lentils (or other pulses) or potatoes will thicken it, while adding more water or stock will make it thinner. (If using lentils, add salt *after* they are cooked, or they will take ages to soften.) Once you have followed a few recipes you will quickly see how to make your own soups any way you like them.

Chicken noodle soup

1 onion   1 clove garlic
2 chicken joints, cut into pieces   50 g (2 oz) Chinese-style noodles
175 g (6 oz) Chinese cabbage, chopped

Fry the onion and garlic in a saucepan until transparent. Add the pieces of chicken and cover with water. Bring to the boil and season with salt and pepper. Cover and simmer for about 1 hour. Remove the chicken bones and skin and continue boiling to reduce the liquid by about half. Add the noodles and cabbage, simmer for a few minutes, and serve.

Potato and leek soup

25 g (1 oz) butter or margarine   1 chicken or vegetable stock cube
3 leeks, washed and sliced   3 large potatoes, peeled and chopped
1 litre (1¾ pints) water

Melt the butter in a saucepan and fry the leeks and potatoes lightly with the lid on the pan for about 20 minutes. Dissolve the stock cube in some boiling water, then make up to about 1 litre (1¾ pints), pour over the vegetables and simmer for another 10 minutes, or until cooked. Season as necessary.

Celery soup

1 head celery, washed and chopped   300 ml (½ pint) water
150 ml (¼ pint) milk   1 clove garlic, crushed
50 g (2 oz) red lentils

Put all the ingredients into a saucepan, and simmer until soft. Liquidise, and add seasoning as necessary.

Onion soup

4 large onions, finely sliced   50 g (2 oz) butter or margarine
1 litre (1¾ pints) good flavoured stock

Melt the butter in a saucepan, and fry the onions and garlic until they start to turn colour, then pour in the stock. Bring to the boil, season as necessary, and simmer gently for about 45 minutes.

Cream of carrot soup

400 g (1 lb) carrots, thinly sliced   200 g (½ lb) tomatoes (chopped),
1 litre (1¾ pints) stock   or 1 tin

50 g (2 oz) butter or margarine   250 ml (½ pint) milk
chopped parsley

Melt the butter in a saucepan, and cook carrots gently for a few minutes, stirring occasionally. Add tomatoes and cook for another few minutes. Pour in the stock, season as necessary, and simmer until the carrots are soft – about 45 minutes. Liquidise. Reheat when needed, adding hot milk, and serve sprinkled with chopped parsley.

Lentil soup

a mug of red lentils
1 clove garlic, crushed or chopped
1 litre (1¾ pints) water

2 small onions
2 teaspoons Marmite
any leftover cooked chopped
    potatoes or carrots (optional)

Cook the finely chopped onions and garlic in oil in a saucepan until soft. Add the lentils and water and bring to boil. Simmer until lentils are soft (about 20–30 minutes), then add seasoning, Marmite and chopped vegetables.

Oxtail soup

1 oxtail (usually bought from butcher ready cut up and boned)
onions
stock

Cook oxtail for an hour or two (it is more economical to put it in a slow oven in an ovenproof casserole when you are cooking something else). Remove the oxtail, and when cool skim off the fat. Fry onions until they turn a light brown, add oxtail stock and cook together for about 15 minutes. Season as necessary. Pressure cooking cuts down cooking time considerably.

Bean and tomato soup

8 butter beans or tin of butter beans or tin red kidney beans
2 onions
tin of tomatoes

If using dried butter beans, soak them overnight. Cook onions in saucepan in oil, butter or margarine, add tomatoes and beans, and about 1 litre (1¾ pints) water. Simmer very gently until beans are tender (or for about 10 minutes if using tinned butter beans or kidney beans). Season as necessary.

Leek and carrot soup

2 large carrots, diced   1 litre (about 1¾ pints) stock or water
4 leeks, chopped   25 g (1 oz) butter or margarine
chopped parsley

Sauté leeks and carrots together in butter or margarine in a sauce-pan until slightly browned. Add stock or water, cover pan and cook gently for 30–40 minutes until vegetables are cooked. Serve as it is for a thin soup, or liquidise for a thick soup. Sprinkle with chopped parsley.

Main dishes

The recipes in this section are just a tiny selection of what you could eat at a main meal. They are inexpensive, easy to shop for, quick to prepare, nutritious, and most have a good fibre content. There is nothing magical about them – you can adapt them according to your preferences, and to what you have in the kitchen cupboard.

Chicken parcels

For each person you will need:

1 chicken portion   lemon and thyme stuffing (from a packet)
1 large potato   1 or 2 wide rashers of bacon

Make up a small quantity of lemon and thyme stuffing (about 1–2 tablespoons per person) and spread over chicken portion. Wrap a rasher of bacon around it. Cut potato in half lengthways, and place one half on each side. Sprinkle with salt and pepper. Wrap all round with foil, turn over edges of foil to seal well, and cook for about an hour at 180°C (350°F, gas 4).

Quick chicken casserole

1 chicken portion per person
1 tin of mushroom soup
some sliced vegetables, such as carrots, courgettes, celery, or leeks
2 lemon quarters

Place chicken portions in casserole dish, cover with mushroom soup and sliced vegetables. Add lemon quarters. Cook for about 30 to 40 minutes at 180°C (350°F, gas 4). Remove lemon before serving.

Cheesy leeks (or any other vegetable)

enough leeks or other vegetable per person
25 g (1 oz) butter or margarine 25 g (1 oz) flour
250 ml (½ pt) milk some grated cheese
Worcestershire sauce (optional)

Wash the vegetables, cut into fairly large portions and place in an ovenproof dish. Make cheese sauce: melt butter or margarine, stir in flour and slowly add milk, stirring until quite smooth. Add enough grated cheese to give a good flavour, and (optional) add a few drops of Worcestershire sauce. Pour sauce over vegetables, sprinkle some more grated cheese on top, and cook for about 30 minutes at 180°C (350°F, gas 4).

Pasta

Pasta is cheap, nutritious and easy to prepare. Wholewheat pasta is higher in fibre than ordinary (white) pasta. Allow 75–100 g (3–4 oz) per person, more if you are very hungry. Pasta comes in a wide range of shapes, and you can serve it with any number of different sauces. Cooking times differ according to the make and variety, so check on the packet.

Some ideas for sauce are:

onion and tomato chicken liver and tomato
mushroom and tomato mince
mushroom, garlic and yogurt tomato and herbs
tuna fish and mushroom prawn and tomato

Pasta also makes a very good salad. Allow about 50 g (2 oz) per person and add anything you like, with a light dressing:

cubes of Cheddar cheese thinly sliced leeks
pieces of tuna fish chopped hard-boiled eggs
red, green and yellow peppers mushrooms, cooked or raw
any leftover cold meats nuts
sliced courgettes chopped oranges or apples

If you can't eat wheat, your local supermarket or health food shop may stock wheat-free pasta. Or contact one of the suppliers of wheat-free products (see 'Useful addresses').

Rice

Rice is one of the few foods that seems to disagree with almost nobody. Allow about 75 g (3 oz) per person for a main dish and about 50 g (2 oz) per person for a salad.

Simple risotto

1 onion, chopped
100 g (4 oz) rice (this recipe uses white rice, so if using brown rice you will need more liquid, and a longer cooking time)
50 g (2 oz) grated cheese
400 ml (¾ pint) chicken stock, or 1 chicken stock cube dissolved in about 400 ml (¾ pint) boiling water
a handful of currants
about 75 g (3 oz) leftover cooked chicken or ham, diced

Fry the onion lightly until transparent, stir in the rice and cook for a few minutes. Carefully add the stock, and simmer gently until all the liquid has been absorbed and the rice is just cooked (white rice takes 15–20 minutes, brown rice 30–40 minutes). Add the currants, diced meat and grated cheese, mix quickly together, heat through for about 5 minutes, and serve at once.

Rice salad

Cook the rice according to the instructions on the packet and allow to cool. While still warm, fluff up with a fork if it looks like sticking together (using American-style easy-cook rice gets over this problem). When cold you can add almost anything to it, with or without a dressing.

Stuffed vegetables

You can stuff peppers, marrows, or even giant mushrooms.

For peppers, remove the seeds, and blanch in boiling water for about 2 minutes to reduce the strong taste. Marrows should be cut in slices about 2.5 cm (1 in) thick, with the skin peeled off if it is very coarse but not otherwise. Fill with a stuffing of any combinations of:

rice	mushrooms
mince	peas
diced cooked chicken or ham	tuna
nuts	finely chopped leeks and celery

or anything else you can think of, or have left over. Place in a well-greased oven dish, cover and cook until tender.

Pancakes

You can eat pancakes on their own, or stuffed with anything – meats, vegetables, in a sauce or not, as you wish.

A recipe for those who can eat wheat:

100 g (4 oz) plain flour
a pinch of salt
2 eggs
250 ml (½ pint milk) (you can replace up to 50 or 100 ml (2 or 3 fl oz) of the milk with water if you prefer)
2 tablespoons melted butter or margarine

Sieve the flour and salt into a mixing bowl. Make a well in the middle, and break the eggs into it. Beat well, gradually incorporating the flour into the eggs. Add the milk (or milk and water), and beat well until a nice smooth mixture – any lumps will disappear as you continue to beat. The mixture should end up with the consistency of thin cream. Put a very small knob of butter or margarine into a frying pan and allow it to thinly cover the whole base of the pan. Pour into the pan about three-quarters of a ladleful (about 2 tablespoons) of the batter mixture, swirl the pan around quickly so that the mixture quickly spreads over the base of the pan, and cook for about a minute on each side. When the pancake is cooked it should turn easily. You may find the first pancake is not too successful, but the rest should be fine.

Two pancake recipes for those who can't eat wheat:

50 g (2 oz) gluten-free self-raising flour   WF
1 egg
150 ml (¼ pint) skimmed milk

Put the flour into a basin with the egg and mix to a stiff paste. Add the milk, a little at a time, beating it in after each addition. Beat well and it is ready to use.

25 g (1 oz) buckwheat	25 g (1 oz) rice flour WF
50 g (2 oz) gluten-free cornflour	1 egg
150 ml (¼ pint) milk	

Mix the buckwheat, rice flour and cornflour together in a bowl with a little salt. Add the egg and milk, stir well, and leave to stand for 15 minutes. Then stir again and it is ready to use.

Fish

Fish is a much underrated dish. It is quick and easy to prepare, and most nutritious. It can be grilled, baked, poached or cooked in foil. Choose fresh fish if you can, and your fishmonger will tell you how to cook it if you are uncertain; the internet provides plenty of information on cooking fish.

Try to have fish at least once a week – your insides will thank you. Some ideas are:

* trout, herring or mackerel, grilled or baked with a little butter or margarine on top;
* plaice, dabs or dory, gently fried in a little butter or margarine;
* cod, halibut or haddock steaks baked in the oven, or cooked in a 'parcel' of foil;
* smoked fish (kippers or smoked haddock, for example) cooked in the oven with a very little water to stop them becoming dry.

Vegetables

Be adventurous! You really don't need to exist on chips, baked beans, frozen peas and tinned sweetcorn; there are a whole lot of other vegetables out there – these, for example:

artichokes	kale
beans (French, runner, broad)	leeks
beetroot	mushrooms
broccoli	onions
brussels sprouts	parsnips
cabbage	peppers
carrots	spinach
cauliflower	spring greens
celery	swedes
courgettes	

You don't need to boil them to death, either. You can steam them (in a cheap steamer that fits in a saucepan, available in most hardware shops), bake them in the oven, braise them gently in a little butter or margarine in a covered ovenproof dish, serve them chopped with butter and ground black pepper . . . almost any way you can think of.

For example, aubergines can be chargrilled on a gas ring or under a grill or, in summer, on a barbecue. They're delicious with salt, olive oil and lemon juice, or you can make baba ghanoush, a dip to enjoy with fresh vegetables or flatbreads.

Baba ghanoush

There are variations galore of this popular dish, but here are some guidelines to start with.

Cut two or three aubergines in half or in thick, chunky slices, depending on how large they are. Pierce the skins with a fork. Grill over a gas flame until the skins become scorched and blackened, or place under the grill. When the flesh is soft, scrape off the charred skin and whisk, blend or mash with a fork, adding one or two crushed garlic cloves, two or three heaped tablespoons of tahini paste, plenty of olive oil, and lemon juice, salt and pepper to taste.

If you have an unappetising assortment of cold leftover vegetables lurking at the back of the fridge, try the following ideas.

Stir-fry vegetables

Use any leftover vegetables, chopped fairly small, to which you might add some beansprouts, cooked macaroni or spaghetti, and tofu cut into small cubes. Fry them all together in a small amount of oil until heated through, adding a few drops of tamari to enhance the flavour.

Vegetable pie

Fry all the leftover vegetables together for a minute or two, put them into an ovenproof dish, cover with a cheese sauce, and top with pastry (frozen puff pastry is ideal). Cook until the pastry is a light brown colour, following the cooking instructions on the packet of pastry.

Salads and salad dressings

Salads are ideal to add to any main dish, or to eat on their own, or to take to work in a plastic container. Here are some suggestions for basic salads, which you can have with salad dressing or mayonnaise, or on their own:

- kidney bean, onion and chopped ham
- diced beetroot, grated carrot and watercress
- cottage cheese, nuts and tinned peaches
- watercress, celery, apple and apricot
- homemade coleslaw with anything you like
- pasta, tuna and cheese (for other pasta salad ideas, see page 51)
- diced cooked potato, tuna and peas
- cauliflower, sliced leeks and kidney beans
- mixed beans – kidney beans, butter beans, sliced French beans
- grated carrot and sultana
- sliced courgettes, French beans and apple
- salad of sprouting seeds – beansprouts, alfalfa, etc.
- sliced tomato and onion with black pepper
- white cabbage with raisins and peanuts
- rice-based salads, adding anything you like
- cooked green lentils, with raw onions, mushrooms and grated carrot

. . . stop when your imagination runs out!

Salad dressings

As with salads themselves, you can be infinitely creative with the dressings. Here are just a few ideas:

- Yogurt with a teaspoon of dried mint and a tablespoon of lemon juice;
- 2 tablespoons vinegar, 4 tablespoons sunflower oil, 1 teaspoon dried mustard (or 1 teaspoon made mustard), 2 teaspoons sugar, salt and pepper;
- 2 tablespoons apple juice, 3 tablespoons sunflower oil, 1 teaspoon sugar, salt and pepper;
- 2 tablespoons lemon juice, 3 tablespoons sunflower oil, 1 tablespoon honey, seasoning;
- yogurt with wine vinegar and garlic;
- tofu with garlic and lemon juice;
- tofu with oil, lemon juice, honey and dry mustard.

Bread, dough and pastry

If you can eat wheat, you should have no problem finding wholemeal bread and flour. If you can't eat wheat, here are some recipes for non-wheat bread, dough and pastry.

The first few recipes are made using a gluten-free flour such as Doves Farm flours (see 'Useful addresses'), and the last ones use rice flour, millet flour and buckwheat. If you experiment with different sorts of non-wheat flour, you should soon find the one that suits you best.

A certain amount of trial and error will probably be needed to obtain best results in individual ovens. You may need to experiment with the exact amount of liquid you use, adding a little extra if need be.

White bread (from Glutafin)   WF

500 g (whole packet) Glutafin Gluten Free Bread Mix
10 g (whole sachet) yeast (enclosed with mix)
350 ml (12 fl oz) hand-hot water (use 1/3 just boiled and 2/3 cold for hand-hot)
1 tbsp (15 ml) vegetable oil (light/mild olive oil recommended)

Combine bread mix and yeast together with a fork. Add the water and oil and stir with the fork to make a smooth stiff batter. Spoon into a lightly greased 2 lb loaf tin. Smooth surface with the back of a dessert spoon dipped in water. Cover with oiled cling film or another inverted bread tin and prove in a warm place until the batter rises to the top of the tin. Remove film or inverted tin and bake for approximately 35 minutes at 220°C (425°F, gas 7) until golden. Allow to cool before cutting.

From <www.glutafin.co.uk/recipe>.

Brown bread (from Glutafin)   WF

Make in the same way as the white bread above, but use brown gluten-free flour.

Both these recipes can also be used to make dough for a pizza base. Instead of putting the newly mixed dough into a loaf tin, roll it out on a floured worktop until it looks like thick pastry. Transfer to a baking sheet. Cover with whatever ingredients you like – sliced tomatoes, mushrooms, ham, anchovies, etc. – sprinkle with cheese and herbs then leave to rise in a warm place for just 10 minutes. Put into the oven at 220°C (425°F, gas 7) on the top shelf for 12–15 minutes and serve hot.

Warm Italian flatbread (from Glutafin)

350 g (12 oz) Glutafin Select Gluten Free Multipurpose White Mix
1½ x 5 ml teaspoon dried yeast (in sachet with mix)
½ x 5 ml teaspoon caster sugar

2 x 5 ml teaspoon skimmed milk powder
¼ x 5 ml teaspoon salt
300 ml (11 fl oz) hand-hot water (use 1/3 just boiled and 2/3 cold for hand-hot)
1 x 15 ml tablespoon mild olive oil

There are a number of gluten-free fillings and toppings you can add in the flatbread, like sundried tomatoes, olives or rosemary, or simply choose your favourite ingredients.

Combine the Glutafin Gluten Free Flour Mix and yeast together in a medium-sized bowl with a fork. Stir in remaining dry ingredients. Add water and oil and stir to make a smooth stiff batter. Combine chosen gluten-free filling ingredients together and stir half of the combined mixture into the bread batter. Spoon into a 23 cm/9 inch greased square baking tin, and top with the remaining filling. Cover with oiled cling film

Leave to prove in a warm place for 45 minutes until the mixture has risen by half. Remove film and bake in a pre-heated oven for approximately 30 minutes at 200°C (400°F, gas 6) until the bread is crisp and golden in colour.

Serve warm in squares. Once cool, store in an airtight container in a cool place for up to three days. Warm before eating for best results.

Gluten Free Wheat Free option   WF

Use 375 g (13 oz) of Glutafin Gluten Free Wheat Free Multipurpose White Mix and all ingredients except caster sugar and skimmed milk powder. Proving time is 1 hour.

If you have any left over, serve the bread with dipping oil. Combine balsamic vinegar, a pinch of mixed dried herbs and olive oil and serve in a small bowl accompanied by squares of warm flatbread. This flatbread is also delicious served with hummus (see p. 46) or any savoury dips.

This bread is suitable for home freezing. Seal in a freezer bag and use within a month. Best warmed through before serving.

From: <www.glutafin.co.uk/recipe>.

Fibre oven-baked loaf (from Glutafin)   WF

250 g (9 oz) Glutafin Gluten Free Wheat Free Fibre Bread Mix
1 x 5ml teaspoon dried yeast (in sachet with mix)
250 ml (9 fl oz) hand-hot water (use 1/3 just boiled and 2/3 cold for hand-hot)
2 x 5ml teaspoon vegetable oil, plus extra for greasing and brushing

Combine the Fibre Bread Mix and yeast together in a medium-sized bowl using a fork. Add the water and oil and stir together to make a smooth stiff batter.

Spoon batter into a well-greased, non-stick 450 g (1 lb) bread tin. Smooth the surface with the back of a dessertspoon dipped in water. Brush with the oil and cover tin with cling film. Prove in a warm place until the batter reaches level with the top of the tin. Remove film and bake for approximately 35 minutes at 220°C (425°F, gas 7) until golden. The bread is best eaten within two days.

From: <www.glutafin.co.uk/recipe>.

Shortcrust pastry   WF

225 g (8 oz) gluten-free plain flour
2 pinches salt
75 g (3 oz) soft margarine 5 tablespoons cold water

Mix the flour with the salt in a mixing bowl. Rub in the margarine until the mixture resembles breadcrumbs. Add the water and mix to a sticky paste (the water releases the binder from the flour). Knead gradually, adding only a very small amount of extra flour, until one ball of dough has formed and the bowl is clean.

This pastry is easiest to use for small items that can be cut out of rolled-out dough and lifted off the worktop with a spatula. For larger items such as pies and pastries, the dough should be rolled out between sheets of silicone paper (often called baking parchment paper) or greaseproof paper. The top paper is then peeled off and the pastry turned upside down over the dish allowing the backing sheet to peel off. Any excess should be trimmed off with a knife and any breaks can be pressed together. The pastry lid should then be rolled out in the same way and dropped on to the filled pie.

If preferred, the bottom part of pies can be pressed out with the fingers until the dish is neatly lined.

Bake for about 20 minutes at 220°C (425°F, gas 7).

Crispbreads – makes about eight large crisp biscuits   WF

15 g (½ oz) rice bran   a pinch salt
90 g (3½ oz) gluten-free plain flour   25 g (1 oz) soft margarine
3 tablespoons cold water

Put the rice bran into a bowl with the salt and flour. Mix well. Add the margarine and rub in with the fingers until mixture resembles fine breadcrumbs. Add the cold water and mix into one large lump of dough. Roll out using more flour into a thin sheet of dough. Use a knife to cut into about eight rectangles, or 16 smaller rectangles if preferred. Lift on to ungreased baking sheet with a spatula and prick all over with a fork. Bake for approximately 15 minutes at 230°C (450°F, gas 8). Remove from the baking sheets with a spatula. Leave to cool and crisp on a wire rack.

When cold, store in an airtight container. Use instead of bread, spread with butter or margarine, or top with ingredients of your choice to make an open sandwich.

Banana bread (with gluten-free flour)   WF

175 g (6 oz) gluten-free self-raising flour   50 g (2 oz) ground rice
a pinch salt   50 g (2 oz) soft margarine
50 g (2 oz) soft brown sugar   1 egg, beaten
rind of 1 lemon, finely grated   1 medium-sized banana, mashed

Put the flour, ground rice and salt into a bowl. Mix well. Rub in the margarine with the fingers. Stir in the sugar, egg, lemon rind and mashed banana. Spoon into a greased and floured small loaf tin. Bake for 45 to 50 minutes at 180°C (350°F, gas 4) until light brown. Turn out of the tin and leave to cool on a wire rack. When cold serve thickly sliced and spread with butter or margarine. Store in a polythene bag and eat within two days.

Buckwheat loaf   WF

1 tablespoon dried yeast   50 g (2 oz) maizemeal
1 teaspoon brown sugar   25 g (1 oz) soya flour
150 ml (¼ pint) warm water   25 g (1 oz) buckwheat flour
75 g (3 oz) potato flour   ½ teaspoon salt

Mix the dried yeast, sugar and water and leave in a warm place for 15 minutes. Sift the flours into a bowl and add the salt. Stir the yeast and liquid mixture and pour onto the flour mixture. Beat well with a wooden spoon to get rid of the lumps and to give a creamy consistency. Pour into a 450 g (1 lb) loaf tin and leave to stand for 5 minutes. Bake at 180°C (350°F, gas 4) for about 1 hour until well risen and crusty. Remove from the tin and bake upside down for a further 10 minutes. Turn out onto a wire rack to cool.

Date and walnut loaf   WF

225 g (8 oz) chopped dates   1 teaspoon bicarbonate of soda

1 pinch salt   300 ml (½ pint) hot water
1 teaspoon wheat-free baking powder (see page 62)
280 g (10 oz) rice flour   120 g (4 oz) margarine
60 g (2 oz) shelled walnuts, chopped
120 g (4 oz) soft brown sugar   1 egg

Place dates, bicarbonate of soda and salt in a bowl and pour the hot water over the top. Leave to cool. Sift the flour with the baking powder twice. Rub the margarine into the flour. Drain the dates and mix them into the flour along with the walnuts and sugar. Beat the egg and add to the flour mixture. Grease a 900 g (2 lb) loaf tin, fill with the mixture and bake for 1½ hours at 180°C (350°F, gas 4). Turn out on to a wire tray to cool. Currants or raisins can be substituted for dates. This loaf cuts much better if left for a day.

Simple banana loaf (with millet flour)   WF

200 g (7 oz) millet flour
2 teaspoons wheat-free baking powder (see page 62)
½ teaspoon bicarbonate of soda   75 g (2½ oz) margarine
135 g (4½ oz) caster sugar   4 ripe bananas, mashed
2 eggs

Sift the millet flour, baking powder and bicarbonate of soda together. Rub in the margarine until well mixed. Add the sugar and bananas. Mix well. Beat the eggs and add them to the other ingredients. Mix again. Grease a 900 g (2 lb) loaf tin with margarine. Turn mixture into the tin, and bake for 1 hour at 190°C (375°F, gas 5). Turn out on to a wire rack to cool.

Chapatis (makes four)   WF

2 heaped tablespoons gluten-free flour
a pinch salt
3 teaspoons sunflower oil
exactly 2 tablespoons cold water
sunflower oil for frying

Put all the ingredients into a bowl and mix to a paste. Use more of the flour to knead. Divide into four and roll out thinly, using more flour. Heat, but do not grease, a griddle or heavy-based frying pan. Cook the chapatis on both sides for about 1 minute or until crisp. When ready to use, heat a little oil in a frying pan. Fry quickly on both sides for a few seconds, just to recrisp them. Stack on a plate after draining on kitchen paper. Serve with curry and rice.

If you can eat wheat, chapatis can be made using special chapati flour, in which case you should follow the directions on the packet. You can also use this recipe:

200 g (7 oz) wholemeal flour   140 ml (5 fl oz) warm water
½ teaspoon salt

Mix the flour and salt together, add the warm water and mix to a dough. Knead well, then cover and leave for 30 minutes. Break off a piece of dough the size of a large walnut, and using plenty of flour, roll into a circle about 20 cm (8 inches) in diameter. Thoroughly heat a large, slightly oiled frying pan and cook the chapati until it is brown; turn it over and cook on the other side. Repeat with the rest of the dough. Keep the chapatis warm until ready to serve.

Tortillas (makes about six)   WF

110 g (4 oz) cornmeal   cold water to mix

Put the cornmeal into a bowl and gradually add water to make a firm dough, while you mix. Break off pieces of the dough and roll them out as thinly as you can, between sheets of greaseproof or silicon paper. Heat a griddle or heavy-based frying pan and cook the tortillas for 1 minute on each side, without greasing. Use instead of bread, with meals.

Tacos   WF

Make as for tortillas and, while still warm from cooking, fold lightly in half. Leave to cool on a wire rack. Use to stuff with salad vegetables or any sandwich fillings. There are lots of ideas on pages 44 and 56.

Homemade wheat-free baking powder   WF

60 g (2 oz) rice flour   60 g (2 oz) bicarbonate of soda
130 g (4½ oz) cream of tartar

Sift the ingredients together at least three times. Store in an airtight container in a dry place. If using instead of standard baking powder, increase amount by 50 per cent – that is, if a recipe calls for 2 teaspoons standard baking powder, use 3 teaspoons homemade powder.

Cakes and biscuits

This section has recipes for cakes and biscuits that do not contain wheat.

Basic plain cake (you can add various flavourings)   WF

50 g (2 oz) margarine   100 g (4 oz) gluten-free self-raising flour
50 g (2 oz) sugar   1 egg
flavouring of your choice

Grease and flour a 450 g (1 lb) loaf tin. Put all ingredients in a bowl, including the flavouring you have chosen, and mix to a soft creamy consistency. If you think it is too stiff, add a little cold milk. Put the mixture into the prepared loaf tin and bake for the first 25–30 minutes at 190°C (375°F, gas 5), then for another 20–25 minutes at 180°C (350°F, gas 4) to cook the centre. Let the cake cool in the tin for a minute and then turn out on to a wire rack to cool. If you wish you can sprinkle the top of the cake with granulated sugar before you put it in the oven.

Do not overbake this type of cake or it will be too dry. The actual baking time depends on the type of flavouring used:

Orange	add the finely grated rind of one orange.
Lemon	add the finely grated rind of one small lemon.
Ginger	add 1 heaped teaspoon dried ginger.
Chocolate	add 2 heaped teaspoons cocoa.
Spice	add 1 heaped teaspoon mixed spice.
Coffee	add Camp liquid coffee (1 or 2 teaspoons according to taste), or dissolve ½ teaspoon instant coffee in 2 tablespoons boiling water.
Carob	add 2 heaped teaspoons carob powder. Use the shortest cooking time.
Vanilla	add a few drops of vanilla essence or flavouring.

Basic fruit cake mix   WF

50 g (2 oz) sugar   50 g (2 oz) soft margarine
2 eggs   100 g (4 oz) gluten-free self-raising flour
rind of ½ lemon, finely grated
100 g (4 oz) dried fruit – currants, sultanas, raisins, cherries, apricots according to taste

Grease and flour a 450 g (1 lb) loaf tin. Put all the ingredients into a mixing bowl, except the dried fruit. Mix until it is a soft dropping consistency. If it is too heavy, add a little milk and beat again. Stir in the fruit. Sprinkle the top with a little sugar if you wish. Bake for half an hour at 190°C (375°F, gas 5) and then either move the cake down one shelf or lower the heat to 180°C (350°F, gas 4). Bake for another half an hour. Leave to cool in the tin for a minute or two and then turn out on to a wire rack to finish cooling. When cold store in an airtight container. Eat within a week of baking.

Rich chocolate cake   WF

200 g (7 oz) gluten-free self-raising flour   2 level tablespoons cocoa
130 g (5 oz) caster sugar   2 tablespoons treacle
2 eggs   5 tablespoons vegetable oil
5 tablespoons milk

Sift the flour and cocoa into a mixing bowl. Add the sugar and mix well. In a smaller bowl, put the treacle, eggs, oil and milk. Stir for a minute until blended well. Grease two 17.5 cm (7 inch) round sponge tins and flour them. Add the contents of the small bowl to the large one and mix well to form a shiny brown batter. Pour into the two prepared sponge tins. Bake for 45–50 minutes at 160°C (300°F, gas 3). When they are ready the cakes will have shrunk slightly away from the sides of the tins, and when pressed lightly they will spring back. Leave to cool in the tin for a couple of minutes, then turn out on to a wire rack to cool. Sandwich together with butter icing or jam. Store in an airtight container.

Plain biscuits (makes about 20 large biscuits)   WF

225 g (8 oz) gluten-free self-raising flour   50 g (2 oz) soft margarine
50 g (2 oz) sugar   1 egg

Cream the margarine and sugar. Beat in the egg. Add the flour and mix to one ball of dough. Knead, using more of the flour and a little cold water if too stiff. Roll out the dough to about 2–3 cm (1 inch) thick and cut into shapes with cutters or divide up with a sharp knife. Use a spatula to place on ungreased baking sheets. Prick with a fork and bake until pale gold – about 15 minutes at 200°C (400°F, gas 6). Cool on a wire rack. Sprinkle with caster sugar and store in an airtight container.

This is a very useful basic biscuit recipe which can be flavoured, iced, sandwiched, topped etc. You can add the following flavourings:

Coffee   add Camp liquid coffee (1 or 2 teaspoons accord-
                    ing to taste) to the flour, or add ½ teaspoon instant
                    coffee dissolved in 2 tablespoons boiling water.

Spice	add ½ teaspoon mixed spice to the flour.
Cinnamon	add ½ teaspoon cinnamon to the flour.
Lemon	add the finely grated rind of half a lemon.
Orange	add the finely grated rind of one orange.
Chocolate	add 1 heaped teaspoon of cocoa to the flour.

Fruit cookies   WF

25 g (1 oz) polyunsaturated margarine
50 g (2 oz) ground rice   ½ eating apple, finely grated
1 tablespoon brown sugar   3 pinches mixed spice
1 slightly heaped tablespoon dried fruit
grated rind of ¼ orange or lemon

Put margarine and ground rice into a bowl and blend with a fork. Add
the apple, sugar, fruit, spice and rind. Mix with a wooden spoon until
the dough forms one ball. Grease a baking sheet with margarine and
drop spoons of the mixture on to it. Flatten slightly with the back of
a teaspoon or a knife. Bake above the centre of the oven for about
20–25 minutes at 230°C (450°F, gas 8). Allow to cool on the baking
sheet for 2 or 3 minutes and then remove to a wire cooling rack, using
a spatula. As they grow cold the cookies will crisp. Eat within a day
of baking.

Fruit and nut cookies

Make as for fruit cookies, but add 1 tablespoon of chopped walnuts,
almonds or hazelnuts.

Ginger nuts   WF

100 g (4 oz) gluten-free self-raising flour   1 level teaspoon dried ginger
3 pinches powdered cloves (optional)   25 g (1 oz) soft margarine
50 g (2 oz) sugar   ½ a beaten egg
2 tablespoon golden syrup

Put the flour, ginger and ground cloves into a basin and mix well.
Beat the margarine to a light cream. Add the sugar and beat again.
Next, beat in the egg and syrup. Add the dry ingredients and mix to
a very stiff paste. Knead, using more flour, and divide into about 16
balls. Roll each ball between your palms, put onto greased baking
sheets, and flatten out to about 4½ cm (1¾ inch). Bake for about
12–15 minutes at 180°C (350°F, gas 4) until a light golden colour.
Cool on a wire rack. Sprinkle with a little caster sugar and store in an
airtight container.

Desserts

Fruit is a good way of getting dietary fibre, so try to eat plenty. Even if citrus fruits (oranges, lemons, grapefruit and limes) disagree with you, there is still a great range available:

apples	plums
peaches	nectarines
greengages	pears
gooseberries	apricots
raspberries	blackberries
kiwi fruit	melons
grapes	blackcurrants
rhubarb	pineapple
mangoes	guavas
lychees	passion fruit
. . . and many more	

The recipes that follow are all easy to shop for and quick to prepare, and most of them are high in fibre.

Crumble topping for fruit (if you can eat wheat)

150 g (6 oz) flour (or 100 g (4 oz) flour and 50 g (2 oz) porridge oats or All-Bran)
80 g (3 oz) butter or margarine
50–75 g (2–3 oz) sugar

Mix all together in a mixer or food processor until it looks like large breadcrumbs. Sprinkle generously over fruit that is already stewed and sweetened, and cook in a moderate oven for 10–15 minutes until the crumble is a pale brown colour. It is a good idea to make a hole in the topping so that the steam can escape, which prevents the fruit spilling over onto the topping.

Crumble topping for fruit (if you can't eat wheat)   WF

150 g (6 oz) ground rice
50 g (2 oz) sugar
75 g (3 oz) butter or margarine

or

150 g (6 oz) ground rice
50 g (2 oz) cooking almonds or porridge oats
50 g (2 oz) brown sugar

Mix all the ingredients together until they resemble large bread-crumbs, and sprinkle a good layer over stewed fruit. Cook as in the previous recipe.

Banana dessert

You can use almost any other fruits for this dessert.

500 g (1 lb) tofu 1 or 2 ripe bananas
2 tablespoons honey a few drops of vanilla essence or flavouring

Blend all the ingredients together, pour into a bowl, and serve well chilled.

Pancakes

Use the recipes on page 53, and serve with lemon juice and sugar or filled with stewed fruit.

Fruit jelly

Make a jelly according to the instructions, add tinned or fresh chopped fruit, and leave in the fridge to set. If you put some of it into a plastic bowl with a lid, you can easily take it to work (but don't let it become warm, or it will melt all over everything!).

Baked apples

1 baking apple per person sugar or honey to sweeten
filling of your choice

Keeping the apple whole, remove the core, enlarge the hole slightly more, and fill with anything you like, such as:

nuts mashed banana
dried chopped apricots crushed pineapple
sultanas and raisins blackberries
tinned pineapple cubes raspberries.

Put on a flat ovenproof dish, add a small quantity of water, sprinkle with sugar or cover with about a tablespoon of runny honey, and bake in a moderate oven until the apple is just soft – about 30 minutes.

Sliced oranges

allow 1–2 oranges per person small amount of water
sugar

Peel the oranges, slice them, and lay them out in a flat dish. Dissolve about 50 g (2 oz) of sugar in about 200 ml (¼ pint) water and heat until melted; it should taste just pleasantly sweet, not sickly. When cool cover the sliced oranges with the sugar syrup, and serve chilled.

Baked pears

allow 1–2 pears per person   runny honey
lemon juice   ½ teaspoon ground cinnamon or ginger

Cut the pears into halves or quarters, and remove the core. Place in a flat ovenproof dish, and cover with honey, a little lemon juice, and a sprinkling of ground cinnamon or ginger.

Dried fruit compôte

Buy a packet of dried fruit – usually a mixture of dried apples, peaches, apricots and prunes. Leave to soak in water for a few hours until tender (it will take less time if you bring the water to the boil first). Can be eaten cold or heated, with sugar or yogurt, or just as it is.

Yogurt with fruit

Make your own yogurt (see page 45), or buy a large carton of plain yogurt. Add some fresh or tinned fruit, and sweeten with honey.

Fruit brulée

soft fruit such as raspberries, sliced bananas, stewed apples, tinned peaches, or any soft fruit you like
whipping cream
demerara sugar

Place the fruit in an ovenproof dish, cover with whipped cream and a good sprinkling of demerara sugar, and place under a hot grill until the sugar bubbles and melts (but take care it doesn't burn). Serve immediately.

Raspberry whip

400 g (1 lb) raspberries (or any other soft fruit)
280 g (10 oz) tofu
sugar to taste

Cook raspberries in a very little water with the sugar until just soft. Leave to cool. Liquidise in a blender or food processor with the tofu until smooth. Serve chilled.

Instant fruit flan

Buy a ready-made flan case from your grocer or supermarket, sweet-flavoured rather than plain if possible. Fill with stewed fruit, and decorate with cream or yogurt.

Carob whip

15 g (½ oz) cornflour
3 tablespoons sugar
250 ml (½ pint) milk
25 g (1 oz) chopped mixed nuts

15 g (½ oz) carob powder
1 egg, beaten
yogurt or whipped double cream

Mix together the cornflour, carob powder, sugar and egg with enough of the milk to make a smooth paste. Heat the rest of the milk in a saucepan, and when it is almost boiling pour over the carob mixture, stirring all the time. Return to the saucepan, and bring to the boil, stirring all the time. Boil for about a minute, then leave to cool. Fold the yogurt or whipped cream into the cooled mixture, add half the nuts, pour into a serving bowl, sprinkle the rest of the nuts on top, and leave to chill.

Rice pudding

Since the days of Victorian literature, rice pudding has had a bad press, but if you are willing to put childhood memories behind you and rethink your previous judgement, you may have a pleasant surprise.

100 g (4 oz) short-grain rice
75 g (3 oz) vanilla sugar (or sugar and vanilla pod)
850 ml (1½ pints) milk   50 g (2 oz) butter
2 eggs, well beaten   nutmeg to grate

Cook the rice very gently in the milk for about 10 minutes. Add the butter and sugar, stirring carefully. Remove from the heat, allow to cool a little then stir in the beaten eggs. Put the mixture into a well-greased baking dish, sprinkle with nutmeg (freshly grated nutmeg tastes much nicer than ground nutmeg) and bake for 30–40 minutes at 150°C (300°F, gas 2). Serve plain or with jam, golden syrup, maple syrup or honey.

Drinks

There has to be more to life than endless cups of coffee! Herb teas are a good substitute, and you can keep one or two teabags concealed about your person for those occasions when you might be expected to drink coffee. They come in many flavours – peppermint, nettle, strawberry, camomile, apple, orange, lime, etc. – as well as 'daytime teas' to keep you awake, and 'night-time teas' to help you sleep. If you find their taste a bit sharp, add a teaspoon or two of honey.

Ginger beer

15 g (½ oz) fresh yeast
400 ml (¾ pint) water

2 teaspoons ground ginger
2 teaspoons sugar

Mix all together in a jug or bowl and leave for 24 hours. Feed daily with 1 teaspoon of ground ginger and 1 teaspoon sugar. After seven days strain the liquid through muslin or old clean tights, and put the solid residue to one side. Mix the strained liquid with 2.5 litres (5 pints) of cold water and the juice of two lemons. Dissolve 700 g (1 ½ lb) sugar) in hot water, and mix well into the strained liquid. Pour into screwtop bottles, and leave for one week before drinking. Divide the solid residue in half, add 15 g (½ oz) fresh yeast, 400 ml (¾ pint) water, 2 teaspoons ground ginger, 2 teaspoons sugar, and repeat as above. You now have the basis of a lifetime's supply of homemade ginger beer.

Homemade lemonade

1 litre (1¾ pints) water
½ teaspoon citric acid
50 g (2 oz) sugar 1 lemon, cut in pieces

Mix all the ingredients together in a liquidiser or food processor. Strain. Leave to cool.

Tomato juice

carton tomato juice
carton yogurt (or about 100–140 g, 4–5 oz)
200 ml (¼ pint) apple juice
a few mint leaves (if available)

Mix all the ingredients together in a liquidiser or food processor. Serve chilled.

Carob and banana drink

You can substitute any other soft fruit – stewed apricots, raspberries, prunes, stewed blackcurrants, etc.

500 ml (1 pint) milk   2 tablespoons carob powder
2 teaspoons runny honey   1 banana, peeled and sliced

Mix all the ingredients together in a liquidiser or food processor. Serve chilled.

Appendix 1

E numbers

As a general rule, it is a good idea to avoid foods that contain additives. But not all E numbers are 'baddies', and the following hardly ever produce any symptoms:

E100	E161(e)	E308	E415	E508
E101	E161(f)	E309	E416	E509
E120	E161(g)	E322	E420(i)	E515
E140	E162	E336	E420(ii)	E516
E150	E170	E363	E421	E518
E153	E172	E375	E422	E529
E160(a)	E290	E400	E440(a)	E530
E160(b)	E296	E404	E440(b)	E542
E160(c)	E297	E406	E460(i)	E559
E160(d)	E300	E407	E460(ii)	E901
E161(a)	E301	E410	E466	E903
E161(b)	E302	E412	E500	E904
E161(c)	E306	E413	E501	
E161(d)	E307	E414	E504	

The following E numbers may be used on food labels as alternatives to the names of additives.

Colourings (Azodyes), E100 to E180

Serial number	Name of additive
E100	curcumin
E101	riboflavin or lactoflavin
E102	tartrazine
E104	quinoline yellow
E110	sunset yellow FCF or orange yellow S
E120	cochineal or carminic acid
E122	carmoisine or azorubine

E123	amaranth
E124	ponceau 4R or cochineal red A
E127	erythrosine BS
E131	patent blue V
E132	indigo carmine or indigotine
E140	chlorophyll
E141	copper complexes of chlorophyll and chlorophyllins
E142	green S or acid brilliant green BS or lissamine green
E150	caramel
E151	black PN or brilliant black BN
E153	carbon black or vegetable carbon
E160(a)	alpha-carotene, beta-carotene, gamma-carotene
E160(b)	annatto, bixin, norbixin
E160(c)	capsanthin or capsorubin
E160(d)	lycopene
E160(e)	beta-apo-8'-carotenal (C30)
E160(f)	ethyl ester of beta-apo-8'-carotenoic acid (C30)
E161(a)	flavoxanthin
E161(b)	lutein
E161(c)	cryptoxanthin
E161(d)	rubixanthin
E161(e)	violaxanthin
E161(f)	rhodoxanthin
E161(g)	canthaxanthin
E162	beetroot red or betanin
E163	anthocyanins
E170	calcium carbonate
E171	titanium dioxide
E172	iron oxide and hydroxides
E173	aluminium
E174	silver
E175	gold
E180	pigment rubine or lithol rubine BK

Preservatives E200 to E297

These prevent bacteria and fungi from causing decay in food:

E200	sorbic acid
E201	sodium sorbate
E202	potassium sorbate
E203	calcium sorbate

E210	benzoic acid
E211	sodium benzoate
E212	potassium benzoate
E213	calcium benzoate
E214	ethyl 4-hydroxybenzoate
E215	ethyl 4-hydroxybenzoate sodium salt
E216	propyl 4-hydroxybenzoate
E217	propyl 4-hydroxybenzoate sodium salt
E218	methyl 4-hydroxybenzoate
E219	methyl 4-hydroxybenzoate sodium salt
E220	sulphur dioxide
E221	sodium sulphite
E222	sodium hydrogen sulphite
E223	sodium metabisulphite
E224	potassium metabisulphite
E226	calcium sulphite
E227	calcium hydrogen sulphite
E230	biphenyl or diphenyl
E231	2-hydroxybiphenyl
E232	sodium biphenyl-2-yl-oxide
E233	2-(thiazol-4-yl) benzimidazole
E236	formic acid
E237	sodium formate
E238	calcium formate
E239	hexamine
E249	potassium nitrite
E250	sodium nitrite
E251	sodium nitrate
E252	potassium nitrate
E260	acetic acid
E261	potassium acetate
E262	sodium hydrogen diacetate
E263	calcium acetate
E270	lactic acid
E280	propionic acid
E281	sodium propionate
E282	calcium propionate
E283	potassium propionate
E290	carbon dioxide

Antioxidants E300 to E321

These stop fats and oils from going rancid:

E300	L-ascorbic acid
E301	sodium-L-ascorbate
E302	calcium-L-ascorbate
E304	6-O-palmitoyl-L-ascorbic acid
E306	extracts of natural origin rich in tocopherols
E307	synthetic alpha-tocopherol
E308	synthetic gamma-tocopherol
E309	synthetic delta-tocopherol
E310	propyl gallate
E311	octyl gallate
E312	dodecyl gallate
E320	butylated hydroxyanisole
E321	butylated hydroxytoluene

Emulsifiers E322 to E495

These improve texture:

E322	lecithins
E325	sodium lactate
E326	potassium lactate
E327	calcium lactate
E330	citric acid
E331(a)	sodium dihydrogen citrate
E331(b)	disodium citrate
E331(c)	trisodium citrate
E332	potassium dihydrogen citrate
E332	tripotassium citrate
E333	calcium citrate
E333	dicalcium citrate
E333	tricalcium citrate
E334	tartaric acid
E335	sodium tartrate
E336	potassium tartrate
E336	potassium hydrogen tartrate
E337	potassium sodium tartrate
E338	orthophosphoric acid
E339(a)	sodium dihydrogen orthophosphate
E339(b)	disodium hydrogen orthophosphate

E339(c)	trisodium orthophosphate
E340(a)	potassium dihydrogen orthophosphate
E340(b)	dipotassium hydrogen orthophosphate
E340(c)	tripotassium orthophosphate
E341(a)	calcium tetrahydrogen diorthophosphate
E341(b)	calcium hydrogen orthophosphate
E341(c)	tricalcium diorthophosphate
E400	alginic acid
E401	sodium alginate
E402	potassium alginate
E403	ammonium alginate
E404	calcium alginate
E405	propane-1, 2-diol alginate
E406	agar
E407	carrageenan
E410	locust bean gum
E412	guar gum
E413	tragacanth
E414	acacia or gum arabic
E415	xanthan gum
E420(i)	sorbitol
E420(ii)	sorbitol syrup
E421	mannitol
E422	glycerol
E440(a)	pectin
E440(b)	pectin, amidated
E450(a)	disodium dihydrogen diphosphate
E450(a)	tetrasodium diphosphate
E450(a)	tetrapotassium diphosphate
E450(a)	trisodium diphosphate
E450(b)	pentasodium triphosphate
E450(b)	pentapotassium triphosphate
E450(c)	sodium polyphosphate
E450(c)	potassium polyphosphates
E460(i)	microcrystalline cellulose
E460(ii)	powdered cellulose
E461	methylcellulose
E463	hydroxypropylcellulose
E464	hydroxypropylmethylcellulose
E465	ethylmethylcellulose
E466	carboxymethylcellulose, sodium salt

E470	sodium potassium and calcium salts of fatty acids
E471	mono- and di-glycerides of fatty acids
E472(a)	acetic acid esters of monoglycerides and diglycerides of fatty acids
E472(b)	lactic acid esters of monoglycerides and diglycerides of fatty acids
E472(c)	citric acid esters of monoglycerides and diglycerides of fatty acids
E472(d)	tartaric acid esters of monoglycerides and diglycerides of fatty acids
E472(e)	diacetyltartaric acid esters of monoglycerides and diglycerides of fatty acids
E473	sucrose esters of fatty acids
E474	sucroglycerides
E475	polyglycerol esters of fatty acids
E477	propane-1, 2-diol esters of fatty acids
E481	sodium stearoyl-2-lactylate
E482	calcium stearoyl-2-lactylate
E483	stearyl tartrate

In addition there are the *flavour enhancers* E620 to E635, of which the most important is monosodium glutamate, and related additives E620 to E623.

Flavourings do not have E numbers, and do not have to be listed on food labels, but they are used in very small quantities and it is not thought that they are harmful.

Appendix 2

Substitute foods

Bread and biscuits	gluten-free bread, rye bread, rye crispbreads, oatcakes, rice cakes, rice crackers
Wheatflour	rice flour, potato flour, soya flour, rye flour, maize flour, buckwheat, millet, oats, oatmeal, arrowroot, tapioca, sago; sauces can be thickened with tapioca flour, potato flour, ground rice
Wheat-based pasta	pasta made with gluten-free flour, rice, rice noodles, buckwheat spaghetti, potatoes
Breakfast cereals	Rice Krispies, puffed rice, porridge, some makes of muesli
Dairy products	goat's or ewe's milk may be suitable, yogurt may be suitable in small quantities, soya milk (calcium-fortified if possible), Granose margarine, Tomor margarine, kosher spreads, sunflower spreads, clarified butter (ghee)
Potatoes	rice, pasta, chapatis, yams, sweet potatoes, dhal, pulses
Corn	wheat, rye, oats, barley
Yeast (in bread)	soda bread, chapatis, unleavened breads
Yeast (in alcohol)	non-alcoholic drinks
Tea or coffee	herb teas, fruit juices, Barleycup, Bovril, Caro, chicory drinks, vegetable drinks
Chocolate	carob, cocoa
Citrus fruits	almost any other fruit
Corn oil or vegetable oil	sunflower oil, safflower oil, soyabean oil
Tap water	bottled spring water is an obvious substitute, but if you think tap water disagrees with you, you should see your doctor before eliminating it.

Appendix 3

Low-fibre diet for irritable bowel syndrome

Fibre is that part of plant foods that our digestive system is unable to break down. It is found in cereals, fruits and vegetables and any foods containing them. Some people find that too much fibre in their diet can aggravate symptoms of diarrhoea, constipation, bloating, flatulence and abdominal pain. Following a low-fibre diet may help to decrease these symptoms.

The following list of foods will help you to make low-fibre choices in your diet. You will probably only need to follow a low-fibre diet for a temporary period. Try following a low-fibre diet for an initial period of four weeks. You may then find that you can gradually re-introduce some of the higher-fibre foods back into your diet to a level that you can tolerate. Guidance on how to re-introduce fibre is given at the end of this appendix.

If you experience constipation while following a low-fibre diet, you may need to take a non-fermentable fibre supplement. Suitable types are normacol, celevac and linseeds. These should be taken with plenty of fluid. Your doctor or a dietitian can advise you about these.

It is important that you have an adequate fluid intake while following a low-fibre diet. You should aim to have at least eight to ten cups of fluid daily.

Low fibre (suitable)	High fibre (unsuitable)
Meat and fish	
All types	Meat or fish made with wholemeal pastry or breadcrumbs
Dairy products	
Milk – all types	
Cheese – all types without pieces of fruit or nuts	Cheese with large pieces of fruit or nuts
Yogurts – natural or fruit-flavoured	Yogurts with added fibre
	Yogurts with large pieces of fruit, cereal or nuts

Low fibre (suitable)	High fibre (unsuitable)

Dairy products (contd)

Cream
Eggs
Fromage frais

Fats and oils

All types

Cereals and baked products

Low fibre (suitable)	High fibre (unsuitable)
White flour and baked products made with white flour such as white bread and toast, crumpets, pastry, chapattis, poppadums	Wholemeal, brown, granary, bran and soya flours and breads Foods made with these flours High-fibre white breads
White pasta,* spaghetti,* macaroni,* noodles*	Wholemeal pasta Cold pasta
White rice,* couscous, tapioca, sago, cornflour	Brown rice Cold rice
Rice Krispies, cornflakes, Special K, Sugar Puffs, chocolate/sugar-coated cereals	Wholegrain breakfast cereals e.g. Weetabix, All-Bran, porridge, muesli and any cereal with added nuts or fruit
Plain biscuits, e.g. Rich Tea, Morning Coffee, Marie, chocolate chip, chocolate, custard creams, malted milk	Wholemeal biscuits, e.g. digestives, flapjacks, HobNobs. Biscuits containing nuts or dried fruit, e.g. Fig Rolls, Garibaldi
Plain cake, e.g. Victoria sponge, Madeira	Cakes with added fruit or nuts
Plain crispbreads and crackers	Rye and wholgrain crispbreads or crackers Oatcakes

*Rice, pasta and potato should be eaten while still hot. When cooled, these foods become more resistant to digestion, effectively increasing their fibre content.

Fruit

Where possible, avoid skins and seeds. Keep to a maximum of two portions a day. Try to spread fruit throughout the day.

Please note that you can choose to eat more fruits than vegetables or vice versa, providing that your total intake does not exceed four portions.

Low fibre (suitable)	High fibre (unsuitable)
Apples	Dried fruit
Apricot	Bananas
Cherries	Banana chips
Fruit cocktail	Blackberries
Grapefruit	Cranberries
Grapes	Currants
Kiwi	Dates
Lychees	Figs
Mango	Gooseberries
Melon	Loganberries
Nectarine	Prunes
Oranges	Raisins
Peaches	Raspberries
Pears	Redcurrants
Pineapple	Sultanas
Plums	Coconut
Rhubarb	
Satsumas	
Strawberries	
Tangerines	

Vegetables and potatoes

Where possible, avoid skins, seeds and stalks. Keep to a maximum of two portions a day, in addition to potato. Try to spread your vegetables throughout the day.

Low fibre (suitable)		Medium fibre (have small portions occasionally)	High fibre (unsuitable)
Asparagus	Marrow	Avocado	Pulse-type beans such as baked, broad, butter, kidney
Aubergine	Mushroom	Beansprouts	Brussels sprouts
Beetroot	Onion	Green/French/runner beans	Chick peas
Carrot	Pepper	Broccoli florets	Lentils
Celery	Potato*	Cabbage	Peas
Courgette	Radish	Cauliflower florets	Sweetcorn

Low fibre (suitable)		Medium fibre (have small portions occasionally)	High fibre (unsuitable)
Cucumber	Swede	Mange-tout	
Leeks	Tomato	Parsnips	
Lettuce		Spinach	
		Spring greens	
		Sweet potato	

*Rice, pasta and potato should be eaten while still hot. When cooled, these foods become more resistant to digestion, effectively increasing their fibre content.

Miscellaneous

Low fibre (suitable)	High fibre (unsuitable)
Puddings	
Ice cream, lollies, sorbets, jelly, milk puddings, rice pudding, custard, blancmange	Any puddings containing fruits or nuts. Crumbles and other puddings made with high-fibre biscuits or flours
Drinks	
Water, squashes, fruit juices	Fruit juice with bits
Tea, coffee	Fruit and vegetable smoothies
Cocoa, Ovaltine	or milk made with fruits and
Fizzy drinks (please note these are low in fibre but they may increase wind and bloating)	vegetables from the high-fibre list
Fruit and vegetable smoothies made with fruits and vegetables from the low-fibre list and within the daily allowance	
Miscellaneous	
Honey, syrup, lemon curd	Marmalade or jam with bits/peel
Smooth jam, marmalade without pips/seeds	Peanut butter
Marmite, Bovril	Nuts, seeds
Corn-, maize- and rice-based snacks, e.g. prawn crackers, rice cakes, cheese puffs, Rice Krispie cakes,	Tropical and Bombay mix
	Potato crisps*
	Wholemeal/wholegrain savoury snacks

Low fibre (suitable)	High fibre (unsuitable)
cornflake cakes	Cereal bars made with oats, dried
Pretzels	fruit or nuts
Boiled sweets, chocolate, toffee	Confectionery containing fruit
Seasoning, spices	and nuts
Soups, stock cubes	Pickles and chutneys
	Lentil, pea and bean soups

*Rice, pasta and potato should be eaten while still hot. When cooled, these foods become more resistant to digestion, effectively increasing their fibre content.

Example meal plan on a low-fibre diet

Breakfast	Fruit juice (without bits)
	Cornflakes or Rice Krispies with milk
	White bread with margarine or butter
	Shredless marmalade or jam
Mid-morning	Tea, coffee or squash
	Plain biscuit
Lunch	Sandwiches made with white bread or crackers or plain crispbread
	Yogurt
	One portion of fruit (from low-fibre list)
Mid-afternoon	Plain scone or plain biscuit
	Tea, coffee or squash
Evening meal	Meat or fish or chicken or eggs
	One to two portions of low-fibre vegetables
	Potatoes or pasta or white rice
	Milk pudding, jelly or cheese and biscuits
	One portion of fruit (from low-fibre list)
	Squash
Supper	Milky drink
	Plain biscuit

Re-introduction of higher-fibre foods

If, after a four-week trial of the low-fibre diet, your symptoms are improved, try introducing higher-fibre foods gradually back into your diet. Introduce only one type of fibre each week using the list below as a guide. This will enable you to determine the types and amounts of fibre that you can tolerate before provoking symptoms again.

Week 1	Try eating oats such as porridge, flapjacks.
Week 2	Try eating the skins on potatoes and on the low-fibre types of fruit and vegetables: for example, apples, pears.
Week 3	Try having an extra piece of fruit or an extra portion of vegetables from the low- or medium-fibre list. Five portions per day of fruits and vegetables (not including potatoes) are recommended for a healthy diet. (NB: One glass of fruit juice counts as one portion of fruit.)
Week 4	Try replacing white bread with wholemeal or granary bread.
Week 5	Try a higher-fibre breakfast cereal: for example, Weetabix, Shredded Wheat, bran flakes.
Week 6	Try re-introducing fruits and vegetables from the high-fibre lists, such as bananas, dried fruit, peas, sweetcorn. Please remember that these re-introductions give a gradual build-up of fibre in your diet. The aim is to identify a level of fibre that you can take comfortably. For example, you may find that you can eat high-fibre vegetables on days when you do not have wholemeal bread and high-fibre breakfast cereals, or vice versa. If this is the case, try varying the sources of your fibre intake on a daily basis to achieve a varied diet.

Vitamin and mineral supplements

If you are unable to re-introduce any of the high-fibre foods back into your diet, you may need to take a multi-vitamin supplement to ensure you meet your requirements. Please discuss this with your doctor or ask for a referral to a local dietitian who can assess the nutritional adequacy of your diet.

Useful addresses

UK

Allergy UK
Planwell House
LEFA Business Park
Edgington Way
Sidcup
Kent DA14 5BH
Allergy Helpline: 01322 619898
Website: www.allergyuk.org

British Dietetic Association (BDA)
Fifth Floor, Charles House
148–9 Great Charles Street Queensway
Birmingham B3 3HT
Tel.: 0121 200 8080
Website: www.bda.uk.com

The professional association for registered dietitians in the UK. The BDA has a number of food fact sheets on its website. Search for private dietitians at: www.freelancedietitians.org

British Nutrition Foundation
Sixth Floor, Imperial House
15–19 Kingsway
London WC2B 6UN
Tel.: 020 7404 6504
Website: www.nutrition.org.uk

Provides evidence-based information on healthy eating and the relationship between diet, physical activity and health.

British Society of Gastroenterology
3 St Andrews Place
Regent's Park
London NW1 4LB
Tel.: 020 7935 3150
website: www.bsg.org.uk

Coeliac UK (formerly the **Coeliac Society**)
Third Floor, Apollo Centre
Desborough Road

High Wycombe
Bucks HP11 2QW
Tel.: 01494 437278
Helpline: 0845 305 2060
Website: www.coeliac.org.uk

CORE (Digestive Disorders Foundation)
3 St Andrews Place
London NW1 4LB
Tel: 020 7486 0341
Website: www.corecharity.org.uk

Funds research into the entire range of gut, liver, intestinal and bowel illnesses.

Crohn's and Colitis UK (the National Association for Colitis and Crohn's Disease)
4 Beaumont House
Sutton Road
St Albans
Herts AL1 5HH
Tel.: 0845 130 2233 (information)
Website: www.crohnsandcolitis.org.uk

Foods Matter
5 Lawn Road
London NW3 2XS
Tel.: 020 7722 2866
Website: www.foodsmatter.com

A support organization that holds an annual Foods Matter Free From Foods Awards, and publishes a magazine about living with allergies, intolerances, or a 'free-from' diet.

The IBS Network
Unit 1.12 SOAR Works
14 Knutton Road
Sheffield S5 9NU
Tel.: 0114 272 3253
Website: www.theibsnetwork.org

A UK national charity offering advice, information and support. Self-help groups are available, and the organization also publishes a quarterly journal, Gut Reaction, which is free to members.

USA and Canada

American Gastroenterological Association
4930 Del Ray Avenue
Bethesda, MD 20814
Tel.: 301-654-2055
Website: www.gastro.org

This Association is intended mainly for doctors, but it has a good Patient Centre, although it cannot respond to requests for medical advice.

Canada + International
IBS Self Help and Support Group
P.O. Box 94074
Toronto, Ontario
M4N 3R1
Website: www.ibsgroup.org

Canadian Society of Intestinal Research
Gastrointestinal Society
855 West 12th Avenue
Vancouver, British Columbia
V5Z 1M9
Website: www.badgut.org

Hypnosis

www.ibshypnosis.com/IBSclinicians.html
A list of US health professionals offering hypnosis treatment for IBS.

Web pages

FODMAPs
www.shepherdworks.com.au
For information and the latest guidelines about FODMAPs.

King's College London – FAQs about FODMAPs
www.kcl.ac.uk/medicine/research/divisions/dns/projects/fodmaps/faq.aspx

Food Reactions
www.foodreactions.org
Set up by Dr Mario Cassar, formerly a biochemist in the NHS, for people with food intolerance. Provides a forum, information, and sales of enzymes for treating food intolerance.

IBS self-help group
www.ibsgroup.org

Online community offering forums, blogs, information, penpals and an international directory of dietitians knowledgeable about FODMAP.

National Council for Hypnotherapy
www.hypnotherapists.org.uk

Linseeds
www.flaxfarm.co.uk/digestion

Steps for Stress
www.stepsforstress.org

Shows and exhibitions

The Allergy and Gluten Free Show: www.allergyshow.co.uk

Foods Matter Awards: www.freefromfoodawards.co.uk

The Good Digestion Show: www.thegooddigestionshow.co.uk

'Free from' and specialist food stockists and food manufacturers

Most major supermarkets offer wide ranges of special-diet foods and advisory leaflets, and extra information is available on their websites.

Artisan Bread Original (ABO)
Tel.: 01227 771881 (9 a.m. to 5 p.m., Monday to Friday); www.artisan-bread-abo.com
Products: rice-flour bread, also gluten-free and wheat-free bread

Bells of Lazonby
Tel.: 01768 898437; www.bellsoflazonby.co.uk
Products: bread and a wide range of other bakery products

Doves Farm Foods Ltd
Tel.: 01488 684880; www.dovesfarm.co.uk
For organic and gluten-free flour

Drossa UK Ltd
Tel.: 020 3393 0859; www.drossa.co.uk/www.drossa.ltd.com

Products: Pasta, gnocchi, flour/bread/sweet mixes

General Dietary Ltd
Tel.: 020 3044 2933; www.generaldietary.com
Products: Ener-G pastas, breads, bakery sundries, cookies, Communion wafers

Genius Gluten Free
Tel.: 0845 874 4000; www.geniusglutenfree.com
Products: breads

GFF Direct
Tel.: 01757 289200; website: www.glutenfree-direct.co.uk
Products: Feel-free pies, pasties and sausage rolls; Il Pana di Anna flour and pastas; Beiker breads, pastas and desserts; breakfast cereals, soups, drinks

Glebe Farm
Tel.: 01487 773282; website: www.glebe-flour.co.uk
Products: bread/flour/cake mixes

Gluten Free Foods Ltd
Tel.: 020 8953 4444; www.glutenfree-foods.co.uk
Products: Barkat breads, pasta, flour mixes, snacks, biscuits, cakes, cereals

The Gluten Free Kitchen
Tel.: 01969 622222; www.theglutenfreekitchen.co.uk
Products: bakery cakes, puddings and savouries.
For outlets in Ireland, contact Juniper Fine Foods (01387 249333).

Hale & Hearty
Tel.: 020 3405 3134; www.halenhearty.co.uk
Products: sweet and savoury mixes, cereals, pastas, snacks

Infinity Foods
Tel.: 01273 456376; www.infinityfoods.co.uk
Products: wheat-free flour, other whole and vegetarian foods

Innovative Solutions UK Ltd
Tel.: 01706 746713; www.innovative-solutions.org.uk
Products: flours, baking ingredients

Juvela
Tel.: 0800 783 1992; website: www.juvela.co.uk
Products: breads, pasta, pizza bases, flour mixes, crackers, biscuits

Lifestyle Healthcare Ltd
Tel.: 0845 270 1400; http://.gfdiet.com
Products: breads, savouries, pizza, sweet treats

Livwell
Tel.: 0845 120 0038; www.livwell.eu
Products: breads, pastries, cakes

MH Foods
Tel.: 0800 130 3056; www.mhfoods.net
Products: breads, mixes, crackers, cakes, sweet treats

Mrs Crimble's
Tel.: 01256 393460; www.mrscrimbles.com
Products: breads, mixes, crackers, cakes, sweet treats

Nutrition Point Ltd – Dietary Specials
Tel.: 0800 954 1981; www.dietaryspecials.co.uk
Products: breads, pastas, frozen meals, mixes, crackers, biscuits

Nutrition Point Ltd – Glutafin
Tel.: 0800 988 2470; www.glutafin.co.uk
Products: breads, flour mixes, pastas, crackers, biscuits

Orgran
Website: www.orgran.com
Order via Naturally Good Food (Tel.: 02476 541990; www.naturallygood food.co.uk)
Products: pasta, crispbreads, cereals,biscuits, soups, snacks, bread/flour mixes

PGR Health Foods Ltd
Tel.: 01992 581715; www.pgrhealthfoods.co.uk
Products: Rizopia brown rice pastas

Roley's
(Based in Netherlands) Website: www.roleys.com
Products: Bakery, teff flour

Tobia Teff
Tel.: 020 7018 1210; www.tobiateff.co.uk
Products: teff flour and cereals

The Village Bakery
Tel.: 01768 898437; www.village-bakery.com
Products: breads, bakery items

Wellfoods Ltd
Tel.: 01226 381712; www.wellfoods.co.uk
Products: breads, flour, pizza bases, muffins

Online shops

Dietary Needs Direct: www. dietaryneedsdirect.co.uk

Ecodirect Ltd (Republic of Ireland): www.ecodirect.ie

The walk-in shop in Dublin may also be visited between 9 a.m. and 4.30 p.m. on weekdays, but call first as it is extremely busy: Tel.: +353-1-620-5053

Gluten Free Foods: www.glutenfree-foods.co.uk

Gluten Free Shop Ltd: www.gluten-freeshop.co.uk

Simply Free: www.simply-free.co.uk

Wheat and DairyFree.com: www.wheatanddairyfree.com

References and further reading

Braimbridge, Sophie and Jankovitch, Erika (2009) *Healthy Eating for IBS (Irritable Bowel Syndrome): In association with IBS Research Appeal*, London: Kyle Cathie.

Brostoff, Professor Jonathan (no date) *Foods Matter*, available at <www.foodsmatter.com/digestive_conditions_coeliac/ibs_causes_gen/articles/another_perspective.html>.

Brostoff, Professor Jonathan and Challacombe, Stephen J. (2002) *Food Allergy and Intolerance*, Burlington, Mass.: Saunders.

Brostoff, Professor Jonathan and Gamlin, Linda (1998) *The Complete Guide to Food Allergy and Intolerance*, London: Bloomsbury Publishing, third edition.

Dean, Carolyn, and Wheeler, Christine (2009) *IBS Cookbook for Dummies*, London: John Wiley & Sons.

Feinmann, Jane (2009) *Living with Gluten Intolerance*, London: Sheldon Press.

Gazzola, Alex (2005) *Living with Food Intolerance*, London: Sheldon Press.

Green, Wendy (2010) *50 Things You Can Do to Manage IBS*, Chichester: Summersdale.

Greer, Rita (1982) *The Gluten-free and Wheat-free Bumper Bake Book*, London: Thorsons.

Greer, Rita (1987) *Healthier Special Diets*, London: Everyman.

Groves, Barry (2008) *Trick and Treat: How healthy eating is making us ill*, London: Hammersmith Press.

Hunter, Dr John (2007) *Irritable Bowel Solutions: The essential guide to IBS, its causes and treatments*, London: Vermilion.

Hunter, Dr John, Workman, Elizabeth and Woolner, Jenny (2005) *Solve Your Food Intolerance*, London: Vermilion, revised edition.

Klein, K.B. (1988) 'Controlled treatment trials in the irritable bowel syndrome: a critique', *Gastroenterology* 95(1): 232–41.

Lessof, M. H. (1983) 'Food intolerance and allergies', *Quarterly Journal of Medicine* 52(206): 111–19.

Nanda, R., James, R., Smith, H., Dudley, C. R. and Jewell, D. P. (1989) 'Food intolerance and the irritable bowel syndrome', *GUT* 30(8): 1099–104.

Nicol, Rosemary (1989) *Coping Successfully with your Irritable Bowel*, London: Sheldon Press.

Ridgway, Judy (1986) *Wheat and Gluten-free Cookery*, London: Arrow.

Science News (2010) 'Proof that a gut-wrenching complaint – irritable bowel syndrome – is not in your head' (20 August); available at: <www.sciencedaily.com/releases/2010/08/100819141950.htm>.

Shepherd, Sue and Gibson, Peter (2013) *The Complete Low-FODMAP Diet:*

A revolutionary plan for managing IBS and other digestive disorders, New York: Experiment.

Skypala, Isabel and Venter, Carina (2009) *Food Hypersensitivity*, Oxford: Wiley-Blackwell.

Thomson, Peter (2001) *Gluten-Free Cookery: The complete guide for gluten-free or wheat-free diets* (Beginners' Guides), London: Hodder-Arnold, revised edition.

Vickery, Phil (2009) *Seriously Good! Gluten-free cooking*, London: Kyle Cathie.

Whitley, Andrew (2006) *Bread Matters: The state of modern bread and a definitive guide to baking your own*, London: Fourth Estate.

Workman, Elizabeth, Alun Jones, Dr Virginia and Hunter, Dr John (1986) *The Food Intolerance Diet Book*, London: Martin Dunitz.

Workman, Elizabeth, Hunter, Dr John and Woolner, Jenny (2005) *Solve Your Food Intolerance: A practical dietary programme to eliminate food intolerance*, London: Vermilion.

Workman, Elizabeth, Hunter, Dr John and Woolner, Jenny (2012) *The New Allergy Diet*, Ebury Digital (Kindle).

Index of recipes